Earl Mindell, R.Ph., Ph.D., is also the author of

Earl Mindell's Supplement Bible

Earl Mindell's Secret Remedies

Earl Mindell's Soy Miracle Cookbook

Earl Mindell's Soy Miracle

Earl Mindell's Food as Medicine

Earl Mindell's Herb Bible

Earl Mindell's Vitamin Bible

Earl Mindell's

ANTI-AGING
BIBLE

Earl Mindell, R. Ph., Ph.D.

A FIRESIDE BOOK
Published by Simon & Schuster

FIRESIDE
Rockefeller Center
1230 Avenue of the Americas
New York, NY 10020

First Fireside Edition 1996

FIRESIDE and colophon are registered trademarks
of Simon & Schuster Inc.

Designed by Richard Oriolo

Manufactured in the United States of America

1   3   5   7   9   10   8   6   4   2

Library of Congress Cataloging-in-Publication Data

Mindell, Earl.
[Anti-aging bible]
Earl Mindell's anti-aging bible / Earl Mindell.
p.   cm.
Includes bibliographical references and index.
1. Longevity.
2. Longevity—Nutritional aspects.
3. Aging—Prevention. I. Title.
RA776.75.M55   1996
613—dc20   95–38420
CIP

ISBN 0-684-84909-7

The ideas, procedures, and suggestions contained in this book are not
intended to replace the services of a trained health professional. All matters
regarding your health require medical supervision. You should consult your
physician before adopting the procedures in this book. Any applications of
the treatments set forth in this book are at the reader's discretion.

Contents

Chapter 1

Maximum Maintenance, Maximum Health

Of all of the spectacular advances in medicine, science, and technology that have occurred during the past century, the ones that have had the most profound impact on our lives are those that have increased human life span. In 1900, the average life expectancy for an American citizen was forty-seven years of age. Today, as we approach the dawn of a new century, the average life span has increased by more than 50 percent to seventy-six. The fastest growing segment of the U.S. population consists of men and women aged seventy-five and older, a group referred to by gerontologists as the "old old." The number of octogenarians among us continues to grow, and some scientists say that humans may routinely achieve a life span of about one hundred fifteen years; still others contend that biological engineering will extend our life span to one hundred fifty years. A few scientists insist that humans could live to be as old four hundred!

The increase in life span that we have experienced during this century is primarily due to improved sanitation, the elimination of many lethal childhood diseases through vaccinations, and other medical advances such as the development of antibiotics. Rare today, death from infection during childbirth was a leading cause of mortality among women at the turn of the century. Thanks to penicillin and its "wonder drug" offspring, bacterial infections such as pneumonia and strep are no longer life threatening.

Although heart disease is still the leading cause of death in the United States, the mortality rate from heart disease is declining due to better prevention and more aggressive treatments. Although cancer continues to be the second leading cause of death in the United States, the prognosis for at least certain forms of the disease has vastly improved within the past century. We owe a debt of gratitude to the scientists and physicians who have taken us this far. But there are limits to what they have been able to do. Members of the medical establishment readily acknowledge that although we have managed to extend the length of life, in many cases we have done little to improve the quality of life. A recent editorial in a medical magazine lamented the fact that "the ratio of active life to disabled or functionally compromised life has not increased and may actually have diminished during the last quarter of a century" (*Patient Care*, February 28, 1994). In other words, people may be living longer, but they're not living better.

Despite the increase in life span, the perception of aging as a depressing downward spiral of growing wrinkled, growing senile, growing ill, and growing old persists. Indeed, for many of today's elderly, growing older is synonymous with illness. About half of all people over sixty-five are taking multiple medications for a wide variety of ailments. The average older person takes twelve doses of medication daily. For many older people, life is punctuated by visits to the doctor and the hospital. In addition to life-threatening diseases, life-diminishing diseases, such as arthritis, vision problems, memory loss, and sleep disorders, continue to plague the elderly.

This does not have to be the case. Sadly, and ironically, too many people suffer from ailments that are easily prevented or controlled through diet and lifestyle. According to the National Cancer Institute, as many as 35 percent of all cancers may be due to poor diet. Experts estimate that as many as 50 percent of all cases of heart disease might be averted by changes in diet and lifestyle, which themselves would greatly enhance both the quantity and quality of life.

Why and how we age is still very much a mystery. Serious research on aging is relatively new, and only a few scientists are doing concentrated work in this area. Until recently, scientists were disdainful of colleagues involved in aging research, likening it to alchemy or the pursuit of the mythical fountain of youth. However, as the U.S. population has begun to age, interest in the aging process and age-related illnesses has begun to attract greater attention.

Until recently, there was a fatalistic attitude about aging that was shared by both experts and laypeople alike. They believed that there was little they could do to prevent the ravages of aging. Today we know better. There is strong evidence that the downward spiral is not inevitable. For one thing, although they are still in the minority, there is a growing population of "old old" people who are aging well and who have managed to stay active and healthy. We see them on tennis courts, in adult education classes, in the gym, and sometimes still on the job. Researchers have begun to study the lives and lifestyles of these successful agers in the hope of discovering important information that will help us all age well. There is a growing body of research that suggests that with appropriate and timely intervention the downward spiral associated with aging need not happen. Researchers throughout the world are finding new and exciting ways to maintain health and vitality well into old age and innovative ways to prevent some of the common ailments associated with aging. Scientists all over the United States—at Boston's Tufts University, the University of California, Mount Sinai Medical Center in New York, and the University of Texas to name a few—are engaged in research that has generated important information on why and how we age. Here are some of their fascinating findings:

- Vitamins and supplements (antioxidants) may help to protect the body against compounds that may speed up the aging process.
- A handful of foods and supplements may substantially reduce the risk of developing cataracts and macular degeneration, the leading cause of blindness among the elderly.
- An ancient herb and other supplements may help to prevent memory loss and keep us smart and sharp.
- Vitamins and supplements may help to rejuvenate a "tired" immune system.
- Contrary to the popular belief that our muscles grow weaker as we age, it's actually possible, with the right kind of exercise, to build muscle and maintain strength well into our nineties and beyond.
- A supplement widely used in Japan as a treatment for heart disease (and available at natural food stores in the United States) may help to keep an aging heart pumping as strong as a younger one.
- Prostate problems (common among men over fifty) may be prevented or reversed by a combination of diet and supplements.
- The right combination of herbs and supplements can relieve the discomfort of menopause for many women.

Here is more good news: these tools are readily available to anyone who wants to use them. For the first time, we have the power and the knowledge to change our fate and make a real difference in both the quality and quantity of our lives. Although the sooner we start the better, positive changes can produce positive results at any stage of life.

This book will show you how to get started. I will examine the latest research on aging and show how you can use this information to help you live a longer, healthier life. I have compiled a list of the Hot 100 anti-aging substances—foods, vitamins, supplements, herbs, and other compounds—that can help you age successfully. With few exceptions, the vitamins, supplements, herbs, and foodstuffs that I discuss in this book are easily available in pharmacies and grocery and health food stores. I devote separate chapters to the unique aging issues that confront men and women and take a detailed look at the risks and side effects of prescription drugs. Perhaps most importantly, in the chapter "Staying Well: A Guide to Preventing the Common Ailments of Aging," I stress prevention and drug-free approaches to dealing with many problems that can seriously interfere with the quality of our lives.

Finally, I want to stress that the techniques I describe in this book are not a fountain of youth, although they can help us retain our youthfulness. An eighty-year-old who follows my suggestions is not going to look or feel the same as a twenty-year-old. What I am suggesting is that an eighty-year-old can be vigorous, strong, attractive, and full of life. My goal is not to turn back the clock, but to help you be the best fifty-, sixty-, seventy-, eighty-, and even one-hundred-year-old you can be.

Chapter 2

The Hot 100 Anti-Aging Arsenal from A to Z

The anti-aging Hot 100 contains a select group of vitamins, minerals, foods, herbs, and other supplements that can help us live longer, healthier lives. Except for the rare drug or supplement that may be available by prescription only, the anti-aging Hot 100 is available at natural food stores, pharmacies, herb shops, and, in some cases, your local supermarket.

Caution: If you are taking a prescription drug for a medical condition, do not discontinue the drug without first consulting with your physician or natural healer.

1. Acidolphilus
2. Allium vegetables
3. Aloe
4. Alpha-carotene
5. Alpha-hydroxy acids
6. L-Arginine
7. Ascorbic acid (vitamin C)
8. Ashwaganda
9. Aspirin

10. Astragalus
11. Beta-carotene
12. Bilberry
13. Bioflavonoids
14. Boron
15. Bromelain
16. Burdock
17. Butcher's broom
18. Calciferol (vitamin D)
19. Calcium
20. Capsaicin
21. L-Carnitine
22. Centella (Gotu Kola)
23. Choline
24. Chromium picolinate
25. Cinnamon
26. Citrus
27. Club moss
28. Cobalamin (vitamin B_{12})
29. Coenzyme Q_{10}
30. Cranberry
31. Cruciferous vegetables
32. Dandelion
33. Dong quai
34. Echinacea
35. Ellagic acid
36. Fenugreek
37. Fiber
38. Flax
39. Folic acid
40. Fo-ti
41. Gamma-linolenic acid
42. Genistein
43. Ginger
44. Ginkgo
45. Ginseng
46. Glutathione
47. Grapeseed extract
48. Green tea
49. Hawthorn
50. Horsetail
51. Legumes
52. Lemongrass
53. Licorice
54. Lignans
55. Ligusticum
56. Lutein
57. Lycopene
58. Magnesium
59. Melatonin
60. Menadione (vitamin K)
61. Milk thistle
62. Monounsaturated fat
63. Motherwort
64. Niacin (vitamin B_3)
65. Nitrosamine blockers
66. Nucleic acids (DNA and RNA)
67. Oat bran
68. Octacosanol
69. Omega-3 fatty acids
70. Papain
71. Pectin
72. Phytic acid
73. Potassium
74. Propolis
75. Protease inhibitors
76. Psyllium seed
77. Quercetin
78. Reishi mushroom
79. Resveratrol
80. Riboflavin (vitamin B_2)
81. Saw palmetto
82. Schizandra
83. Seaweed

84. Selenium
85. Sesame
86. Solanaceous foods
87. Soybeans
88. Sulforaphane
89. Thiamine (vitamin B_1)
90. Tocopherol (vitamin E)
91. Tretinoin
92. Turmeric
93. Umbelliferous vegetables
94. Vitex
95. Water
96. Wheat bran
97. White willow
98. Wild yam
99. Yohimbe
100. Zinc

Acidophilus

FACTS

Several years ago, a television commercial for a popular brand of yogurt contended that eating yogurt was the key to longevity. The commercial featured several centenarians from an obscure part of rural Russia who had one thing in common: they were all lifelong yogurt eaters. At the time, the premise of the commercial may have sounded a bit far-fetched, but scientists are now discovering that there might be something to it after all.

Yogurt contains *Lactobacillus acidophilus* (commonly known as acidophilus), a so-called friendly bacteria that is used to ferment milk into yogurt and is also present in the gastrointestinal tract. Acidophilus not only aids in digestion, but appears to help keep the growth of yeast, such as *Candida albicans*, in check. *Candida albicans* is the cause of many vaginal yeast infections. In fact, acidophilus is a common folk remedy for yeast infection, but more importantly, recent studies suggest that acidophilus may help the body ward off other infections as well.

Acidophilus is present in yogurt and is also available in capsules or granules.

THE RIGHT AMOUNT

Eat two 8-ounce cartons of nonfat yogurt with active cultures daily. (Be sure the carton specifies *active cultures*.)

Take 2 acidophilus capsules three times daily ½ hour before or after meals.

Mix 1 packet of acidophilus granules in 6 ounces of freshly squeezed juice one or two times daily.

POSSIBLE BENEFITS

Antifungal • Women who are menopausal should take note: the vaginal dryness that often accompanies the drop in estrogen can make you more prone to vaginal yeast infections. A carton or two of yogurt a day may be just what the doctor ordered. Those are the findings of a physician at Long Island Jewish Medical Center who recently studied whether acidophilus is effective against vaginal yeast infections. In her study, the physician instructed women with a history of chronic yeast infections to eat 8 ounces, or 1 carton, of yogurt with live acidophilus cultures each day and compared them to non–yogurt eaters. After 6 months, the women who ate the yogurt had far fewer yeast infections than those who did not.

Immune Booster • As we age, our immune system weakens, making us more vulnerable to infections of all kinds. Eating yogurt daily may help to maintain normal immune function. A researcher at the University of California studied the effects of yogurt with live cultures on the immune system. His findings: people who ate two 8-ounce cartons of yogurt daily had higher blood levels of gamma-interferon, a substance that helps the body to ward off infection. He also noticed that the people who ate yogurt with live cultures also had substantially fewer colds and allergy symptoms than those who did not.

PERSONAL ADVICE

I am frequently asked whether acidophilus capsules are as good as eating yogurt with live cultures. Actually, the capsules and granules provide a more potent form of acidophilus. Sometimes the capsules or granules are preferable, especially if you have a yeast problem or are taking an antibiotic that is wreaking havoc on your digestive system by killing off the friendly bacteria. (Erythromycin is a particular offender.) However, in normal circumstances, eating yogurt is probably good enough. In addition, yogurt offers the added benefit of a hefty boost of calcium, which is needed for strong bones and normal blood pressure and heart function.

Allium Vegetables

FACTS

There are five hundred plants belonging to the genus *Allium*, which include garlic, onions, chives, and scallions. The National Cancer Society is investigating many members of the allium family for their potential cancer-fighting properties. In addition, researchers have found that these special vegetables may be helpful in the prevention and treatment of a wide range of ailments including Alzheimer's disease and cardiovascular disease, two problems that are particularly prevalent among the older population.

THE RIGHT AMOUNT

Use these vegetables liberally in your cooking. Red and yellow onions and shallots have the highest flavonoid content of allium vegetables. (Flavonoids may protect against cancer.)

Fresh garlic should be eaten daily—I prefer to bake or stir-fry it. It has a milder flavor than eating it raw. If you can't stomach the stuff, try using odorless garlic capsules. Take 1 or 2 capsules after each meal daily. Try taking them with an internal breath freshener made from parsley seed oil or chlorella.

POSSIBLE BENEFITS

Alzheimer's Disease • At a 1994 meeting on medicinal foods organized by Rutgers University, French researchers reported on a study involving aged laboratory rats with an Alzheimer's-type disease. The researchers noted that garlic extract appeared to slow down brain deterioration. In addition, the garlic normalized the brain's serotonin system: if the serotonin system malfunctions, it can cause depression. Although this information is exciting, it is not yet known whether garlic would have the same effect on human brains.

Cancer Fighter • Hippocrates, the father of modern medicine, used garlic vapors to treat uterine cancer. Recent studies have shown that people who eat a diet high in allium vegetables—including garlic—have a lower rate of stomach cancer than those who don't. Researchers in China interviewed 564 patients with stomach cancer and more than 1100 people without cancer in a region where the risk for gastric cancer is high. Those with the highest intake of allium vegetables had a 40 percent reduction in risk for gastric cancer.

Garlic and onion are both rich in quercetin and selenium, two "hot" antioxidants that may play an important role in cancer prevention.

Garlic oil contains diallyl sulfide, which has been shown to deactivate potent carcinogens in animal studies. Garlic also stimulates the production of glutathione, a potent antioxidant found in the cells that helps to prevent cancerous changes.

Heart Disease • First-century physician Dioscorides prescribed garlic to treat atherosclerosis, a leading cause of heart disease. Indeed, numerous studies can attest to garlic's positive effects on blood lipids. In a recent study performed at the Clinical Research Center and Tulane University School of Medicine in New Orleans, forty-two healthy adults with total cholesterol levels over 200 milligrams per deciliter were given either 300 milligrams of standardized garlic powder in tablet form three times daily or a placebo. After 12 weeks, those who took the garlic experienced a 6 percent total drop in cholesterol versus a 1 percent decline among those on the placebo. Even better, those on the garlic had a 11 percent reduction in low-density lipoproteins, or "bad" cholesterol, versus a 3 percent drop in the untreated group.

Other studies have shown that people who eat an onion a day can raise their high-density lipoproteins, or "good" cholesterol.

Researcher Eric Block discovered a compound in garlic called *ajoene* that appears to be a natural blood thinner, which may prevent the formation of blood clots that can lead to a heart attack or stroke.

Natural Antibiotic and Antifungal • In the Middle Ages, monks used garlic to ward off plague. Before antibiotics, garlic poultices were used on wounds to prevent infection. In fact, garlic was dubbed "Russian penicillin," because during World War II, when antibiotics were scarce, Russian physicians used it to treat infections on the battlefield. Studies show that garlic has some antibiotic properties and is also one of the strongest natural antifungal compounds, especially against *Candida albicans* (yeast infection).

Anti-inflammatory • Eric Block recently discovered a sulfur compound in onion that in test tube studies blocked the chemical chain of events that lead to asthma and inflammatory reactions.

Food for Thought

Only 9 percent of all Americans eat five or more fruits and vegetables daily as recommended by the National Cancer Institute. According to experts at the National Cancer Institute, as many as 50 percent of all cancers could be prevented by eating the right foods.

Aloe

FACTS

There are more than three hundred species of the aloe plant, and several, including the famous aloe vera variety, have been used since ancient times to heal skin wounds. Aloe gel, derived from the leaf of the plant, is an excellent moisturizer and is a common ingredient in skin creams. Several studies confirm that used externally, aloe can promote healing of minor skin burns and abrasions. Recently, a study performed on animals at Texas A&M University showed that, taken internally, aloe may be a potent immune booster.

THE RIGHT AMOUNT

Aloe gel may be used liberally on the skin as needed. The leaf of the fresh plant is highly effective, but if you don't want to grow your own, aloe vera is available in many different forms at drug stores and natural food stores. Buy only products that are made from pure aloe and that list aloe as a primary ingredient. Many products that claim to contain aloe contain a watered-down version of aloe extract or reconstituted aloe vera.

Aloe, which is used as a treatment for constipation, can cause severe abdominal pain and cramps if taken in large amounts. One tablespoon one or two times daily is recommended. Aloe vera is also available in dry capsule form. Each capsule is equal to 1 tablespoon of the juice.

Caution: Aloe should not be ingested by pregnant women.

POSSIBLE BENEFITS

Wound Healing • Several studies have shown that aloe vera gel can help heal skin irritations and wounds due to radiation burns. At one time, researchers believed that aloe vera promoted healing by sealing in moisture, thus preventing the air from drying out the skin. However, scientists now suspect that there are specific chemicals in aloe vera gel that interact with the skin to speed up the healing process.

Wrinkles   •   Like other moisturizers, aloe gel may give the appearance of younger-looking skin by plumping out dry, fine lines. Thus, the wrinkles don't disappear, but they are less noticeable.

Immune Booster   •   This is one of the newest and most exciting uses of this ancient herb. Researchers at Texas A&M University tested aloe on mice implanted with sarcoma tumors. Mice who had been given aloe vera internally had a 40 percent survival rate. All of the untreated mice died. Interestingly enough, researchers found that it was impossible to implant tumors in mice who had been pretreated with aloe vera. Researchers say that the compound works by stimulating the release of *cytokines*, substances with activate the immune system. Aloe is now being tested on human patients.

Alpha-carotene

FACTS

The carotene family consists of about six hundred naturally occurring compounds found in dark, leafy vegetables and yellow and orange fruits and vegetables. Some of these compounds are potent antioxidants, such as beta-carotene and lycopene. However, only a handful of carotenes have actually been studied for their potential health benefits. Recently, researchers have focused on alpha-carotene, and their findings suggest that it may be as important a cancer fighter as any of its better-known cousins.

THE RIGHT AMOUNT

There is no recommended daily allowance for alpha-carotene. Fruits and vegetables are a rich source of many different carotenes, including alpha-carotenes. For example, about one-third of the carotene mixture in a carrot consists of alpha-carotene. Supplements containing alpha- and beta-carotene are available at natural food stores. Take between 10,000 and 25,000 international units daily.

POSSIBLE BENEFITS

Cancer Fighter • For more than a decade, studies have shown that people with diets rich in green and yellow vegetables have significantly lower rates of cancer than people who don't. Many scientists believe that carotenes are responsible for the reduced cancer risk.

A recent study compared the effects of alpha- and beta-carotene and no carotene on cancer cells in a culture medium. High levels of alpha-carotene stopped the growth of the cancer cells. An equal amount of beta-carotene produced a modest drop in cell growth. However, the cancer cells without any form of carotene experienced explosive growth.

In another study reported in *Cancer Research*, mice were fed a known carcinogen and then divided into three groups. One group of the mice was fed a beta-carotene supplement, a second group was given an alpha-carotene supplement, and the third group was given a placebo. The mice taking the alpha-carotene had a 70 percent reduction in the number of tumors versus those taking the beta-carotene or no supplement at all. From these studies, researchers suspect that alpha-carotene may be a better protector against certain forms of cancer than beta-carotene.

PERSONAL ADVICE

I recommend taking a caretenoid complex along with dark green leafy vegetables and yellow and orange vegetables and fruits. It comes in liquid, tablet, or capsule form. Use as directed.

Alpha-hydroxy Acids

FACTS

Alpha-hydroxy acids (AHAs) are naturally occurring compounds found in foods such as sour milk (lactic acid), grapes (tartaric acid), sugar cane (glycolic acid), apples (malic acid), and citrus fruit (citric acid). For more than a decade, dermatologists have used high concentrations of AHAs (up to 50 percent) for scar removal and facial peels. Today, weaker versions of AHAs are sold in numerous over-the-counter skin care products designed to moisturize and improve the skin. Although they may not be the fountain of youth, for many people, AHAs products can produce noticeable changes in the appearance and quality of their skin.

THE RIGHT AMOUNT

Products range from 2 to 10 percent concentration of AHAs. Most dermatologists consider 5 percent or under to be safe for most people. However, some people may find AHAs irritating at any level, and some may be able to tolerate a higher level. Your best bet is to start out with the weaker products and work your way up. Those with very sensitive skin should stick with the weaker products.

POSSIBLE BENEFITS

Skin Rejuvenator • AHAs have been found to loosen the "cement" binding cells on the skin, permitting the top layer of dead cells to shed more evenly and rapidly, thus revealing smoother, fresher-looking skin underneath. Many studies confirm that AHAs are an effective treatment against extremely dry, flaky skin. They have also been used to treat conditions such as psoriasis. In addition, studies show that these skin products may help erase fine lines and age spots and improve the tone and texture of the skin.

There is some controversy in the medical community over the effectiveness of over-the-counter AHA preparations. The more potent products used by dermatologists are more effective; however, they are also more costly and can cause more skin irritation. Many people, however, find that the milder products are surprisingly effective at a fraction of the cost.

L-Arginine

FACTS

L-Arginine is a nonessential amino acid: since the body produces it on its own, we do not need to get it in food. However, recent studies suggest that L-Arginine may play an important role in maintaining health.

L-Arginine can stimulate the growth and release of growth hormone, which is produced by the pituitary gland. As we age, the level of growth hormone steadily decreases. Some experts believe the decline in L-Arginine production may be responsible for many of the degenerative processes associated with aging.

Good food sources of L-Arginine include nuts, sunflower and sesame seeds, chocolate, popcorn, raisins, and brown rice.

THE RIGHT AMOUNT

L-Arginine is available as tablets and powder. Take 2000 milligrams daily at bedtime, about 2 hours after eating. L-Arginine is often taken in combination with two other amino acids: 2000 milligrams ornithine and 1000 milligrams lysine.

Caution: Do not give L-Arginine to children or to adults with schizophrenia. L-Arginine is reputed to promote herpes,

therefore, people with herpes should not use L-Arginine. Very high dosages can cause deformities of the bones and enlarged joints.

POSSIBLE BENEFITS

Wound Healing • Many studies have demonstrated that L-Arginine supplements can promote wound healing of burns and wounds after trauma such as surgery or injury. If you have been injured recently have undergone surgery, talk to your physician or healer about taking an L-Arginine supplement.

Cancer Fighter • Several studies have confirmed L-Arginine's ability to inhibit the growth of tumors in animals. Studies involving human blood cells show that L-Arginine increased the production of natural killer cells (important immune cells) and other compounds that can thwart the growth of tumors.

Male Infertility • Male seminal fluid contains as much as 50 percent L-Arginine. Several studies have linked a low sperm count to low levels of this important amino acid.

Ascorbic Acid (Vitamin C)

FACTS

If you want to live longer, take your ascorbic acid, or vitamin C. Recent studies suggest that vitamin C supplements (in addition to a diet rich in vitamin C foods) may prevent premature death from heart disease and may even be a more important factor in preventing fatal heart attacks than maintaining a low cholesterol level or eating a low-fat diet.

Vitamin C is also a potent antioxidant and works with other antioxidants in the body to help prevent damage from free radicals that may lead to various forms of cancer.

Vitamin C, a water-soluble vitamin, is necessary for the formation of *collagen*, the substance that binds together the cells of connective tissue. Collagen is also essential for the production of new cells and tissues.

Vitamin C is reputed to be good for colds. In fact, several studies show that although vitamin C can't prevent the common cold, it can lessen a cold's severity by decreasing the histamine level in your bloodstream by up to 40 percent. Histamine causes the runny nose and watery eyes associated with colds and allergies.

Good natural sources of vitamin C include mangoes, kiwi fruit, grapefruit, broccoli, cantaloupe, strawberries, sweet red peppers, sweet potatoes, snow peas, and orange juice.

THE RIGHT AMOUNT

The recommended daily allowance (RDA) for vitamin C is 60 milligrams, for smokers, 100 milligrams. (About half of the U.S. population does not get even 60 milligrams of this vitamin daily.) Studies suggest that the RDA is much too low. I recommend 1000 milligrams daily of calcium ascorbate (the gentlest form of vitamin C for your stomach). Although many people can tolerate up to 10,000 milligrams of vitamin C daily, in some people, excess vitamin C can cause dry nose, diarrhea, excess urination, and skin rashes.

POSSIBLE BENEFITS

Heart Disease • Researchers at the University of California looked at the vitamin C intakes and death rates of more than 11,000 men and women. The study showed a dramatic decline in death from heart disease among men with the highest vitamin C intake, especially among those who took a vitamin C supplement. Merely obtaining the RDA for vitamin C through food did not seem to offer any protection against heart disease. The results were similar among women but less dramatic.

There are several reasons why vitamin C may protect against heart disease. Other studies have shown that vitamin C is particularly effective in intercepting oxidants before they can attack blood lipids. Many researchers believe that when low-density lipoproteins, or "bad" cholesterol, are oxidized, it promotes the formation of plaque, which can cause atherosclerotic lesions in arteries.

Raises Blood Glutathione • Glutathione is one of the most important antioxidants produced in the body. It protects cells from damage inflicted by hydroperoxides (free radicals), a natural by-product of metabolism. Low levels of serum glutathione have been associated with cell damage, depressed immunity, and premature aging. A recent study conducted at Arizona State University showed how glutathione levels fluctuate in humans based on vitamin C intake. People on vitamin C–deprived diets had low levels of glutathione; however, when given a supplement of 500 milligrams of vitamin C, blood glutathione levels bounced back to normal.

Cancer Fighter • Many studies have investigated the association of dietary vitamin C and various forms of cancer. We know from these studies that dietary intake of vitamin C (through food, notably fruits and vegetables) appears to offer some protection against cancers of the lung, cervix, pancreas, mouth, throat, esophagus, colon, and stomach. (In particular, vitamin C may protect against cancers of the stomach because it blocks the formation of nitrosamines in the stomach, which are potential carcinogens.)

There is also some evidence that vitamin C may help to protect against breast cancer, especially in postmenopausal women.

Prevents Cataracts • Cataracts, an opaque covering that can form on the lens of the eye, are particularly common among people over fifty. Researchers at the Laboratory for Nutrition and Vision Research at the U.S. Department of Agriculture's Human Nutrition Center at Tufts University suggest that cataracts may be caused by cellular damage due to oxidation. For example, when vitamin C was added to the diet of guinea pigs, their eyes showed less oxidative damage after exposure to ultraviolet light than in pigs not given vitamin C. In human studies, adults taking antioxidant supplements (including C) were less likely to develop cataracts than those not taking vitamins.

PERSONAL ADVICE

Here's one supplement that everyone should be taking!

Ashwaganda

FACTS

The root of the ashwaganda plant is an important healing herb that is commonly used in Ayurveda, the traditional herbal medicine of India. Ashwaganda is a small shrub that is part of the nightshade family, which includes potatoes, tomatoes, and eggplant.

Although many Western natural healers advise arthritics to avoid eating nightshade plants, in Ayurveda, ashwaganda has long been prescribed to treat arthritis. Recent studies show that ashwaganda may indeed be effective against arthritis and may also be a potent weapon against cancer. In recent years, Ayurveda has become very popular in the West because of its emphasis on the prevention of disease.

THE RIGHT AMOUNT

Ashwaganda teas and other herbal products are available at natural food stores. Ashwaganda is included in many herbal formulas for arthritis. Drink 1 to 2 cups of tea daily, or follow the directions on the package.

Caution: Ashwaganda contains some compounds that may be harmful at very high amounts. Do not exceed the recommended dose.

POSSIBLE BENEFITS

Arthritis • Several Indian studies have confirmed that ashwaganda has anti-inflammatory activity and can help reduce some of the stiffness and swelling associated with arthritis in both animals and humans. In one recent study performed at the University of Poona in Pune, India, forty-two patients with osteoarthritis were given an herbal formula that included ashwaganda and zinc complex. For 3 months, the patients took the herbal formula. Then, after a 2-week period to allow the herbs to wear off, the patients were given a placebo for 3 months. The results: while on the herbal formula, the patients experienced a significant drop in severity of pain and stiffness.

Cancer Fighter • Several animal studies have shown that extract of ashwaganda root can inhibit the growth of tumors in laboratory mice.

Aspirin

FACTS

In 1958 when I started pharmacy school, anyone who would have suggested that aspirin—the wonder drug of the nineteenth century—would be touted as a "hot" anti-aging drug at the dawn of the twenty-first, would have been laughed out of the classroom. However, good old aspirin, chemically known as acetylsalicylic acid, holds great promise for the future as a protector against both cancer and heart disease.

Aspirin is actually a synthetic version of salicum, a natural derivative of the bark of the white willow tree, a longtime herbal remedy for headaches, fever, and arthritis. Until recently, aspirin has been used as an analgesic to treat daily aches and pains. However, recent studies suggest that this drug may be underutilized.

THE RIGHT AMOUNT

To help prevent certain forms of cancer and heart disease, I recommend one baby aspirin (about 81 milligrams) taken every day. Your physician may suggest a higher dose if you are at risk of developing heart disease or certain forms of cancer.

Caution: Do not take aspirin on a regular basis without first checking with your physician. People with bleeding disorders or who are taking blood thinners (e.g., coumadin and heparin) should steer clear of aspirin unless advised differently by their physicians. Aspirin can be very irritating to the stomach and can cause bleeding and ulcers in some people. People on aspirin should be closely monitored by their physicians for gastrointestinal bleeding, or other problems. If untreated, bleeding ulcers can cause severe problems, including death.

POSSIBLE BENEFITS

Heart Disease and Stroke • Will an aspirin a day keep the cardiologist away? There's strong evidence that it just might. Aspirin is a blood thinner, that is, it prevents the clumping together of blood platelets, tiny circulating disks that play a key role in the formation of blood clots. A majority of heart attacks and strokes are caused by blood clots forming in arteries that were already narrowed due to atherosclerotic lesions (deposits of lipids and other cells). By preventing the formation of blood clots, aspirin may play a significant role in preventing heart attacks and strokes. Consider the results of several recent studies.

- A study of 22,000 healthy male doctors given 325 milligrams of aspirin daily for 5 years (the amount in one adult aspirin) had 44 percent fewer heart attacks than those who didn't take the aspirin.
- A study of 87,678 female nurses over 8 years found a 30 percent reduction in risk of first heart attack among women who took 1 to 6 aspirins per week. In this study, the aspirin was not prescribed; rather these women took

aspirin on their own to treat headaches or musculoskeletal pain.

- In yet another study of over one thousand recovering heart patients, at the Multicenter Study of Myocardial Ischemia in New Orleans, those who were not taking aspirin were three times more likely to have a fatal heart attack than those who were on the drug.

Cancer Fighter • Aspirin is an anti-inflammatory. It blocks the formation of *prostaglandins*, hormonelike substances in the body that can trigger an inflammatory response. By quelling inflammation, aspirin can help to relieve the pain of arthritis and bring down a fever. Prostaglandins are also believed to promote the growth of cancerous tumors; therefore, by nipping prostaglandins in the bud, aspirin may indirectly be a potent cancer fighter.

Based on a study of more than 635,000 people performed by the American Cancer Society, those who took aspirin were at significantly lower risk of dying from digestive tract cancers (esophagus, stomach, rectum, and colon). In fact, men and women who took aspirin at least sixteen times a month were 40 percent less likely to die from these cancers than those who did not. The risk was lowest among men and women who used aspirin regularly for 10 years or more.

Astragalus

FACTS

As we age, our immune system becomes weakened, leaving us more vulnerable to infection and disease. A handful of vitamins and herbs may help to keep the immune system functioning at optimal levels, and astragalus may be one of them. For centuries, Oriental healers have used this herb to treat a wide variety of ailments, ranging from diabetes to high blood pressure, and have also prescribed it as an immune booster that strengthens the Wei Ch'i, or defensive energy of the body. Western scientists are now beginning to acknowledge that this herb may indeed have a positive effect on immunity.

Astragalus, which is native to China and Japan, is being studied in the United States as a possible treatment for AIDS, a disease characterized by the breakdown of the immune system.

THE RIGHT AMOUNT

Astragalus is available in capsule form at natural food stores. Take 1 to 3 (400 milligrams) capsules daily.

POSSIBLE BENEFITS

Immune Booster • Research by Dr. G. Mavligit of the University of Texas Medical Center in Houston found that a purified extract of astragalus stimulates T cells (one of the key white cells of the immune system) in healthy animals and helps to normalize the immune systems of cancer patients with impaired immunity due to chemotherapy. Other studies have shown that astragalus can stimulate the production of interferon, a protein produced in cells that fights against viral invasion. In fact, according to one Chinese study, patients given astragalus root developed less colds than patients not given the root; and when they did get a cold, they had it for a significantly shorter amount of time than untreated patients.

Heart Disease • In China, astralagus has been used to treat cardiovascular disease. Animal studies show that this herb can lower blood pressure and may help to prevent heart attacks by improving the flow of blood to the heart.

Beta-carotene

FACTS

Beta-carotene, one of six hundred or so naturally occurring plant compounds in the carotene family, is also known as provitamin A. Some of the beta-carotene we eat is converted to vitamin A as the body needs it. Although beta-carotene is an antioxidant, when it is converted to vitamin A, it loses much of its antioxidant properties.

Of all the phytochemicals, beta-carotene is one of the most widely studied. Numerous studies show that people who eat diets rich in beta-carotene have lower levels of cancer and coronary artery disease than those who don't.

Good food sources of beta-carotene include apricots, sweet potatoes, broccoli, cantaloupe, pumpkin, carrots, mangoes, peaches, and spinach.

THE RIGHT AMOUNT

The recommended daily allowance for vitamin A is 5000 international units or 1000 retinol equivalent. Three milligrams of beta-carotene is equal to 5000 international units of vitamin A. Although vitamin A can be toxic at doses higher than 25,000 international units daily, beta-carotene is not believed to be toxic even at high doses. In fact, many studies used dosages as high as 50 milligrams of beta-carotene without any problem.

Most scientists agree that we need at least 6 milligrams (10,000 international units) of beta-carotene daily; many recommend as much as 14 milligrams (23,333 international units) daily. Most Americans ingest about 2 milligrams (3,333 international units).

Beta-carotene supplements are sold separately. In addition, beta-carotene is included in most antioxidant formulas as well as most multivitamins.

Beta-carotene comes in two forms that vary slightly in molecular structure: all-*trans*- and 9-*cis*-beta-carotene. The 9-*cis* form may be better absorbed by the body.

POSSIBLE BENEFITS

Cancer Fighter • A study presented at the 1994 American Cancer Society Science Writer's Seminar showed that beta-carotene can reverse precancerous sores in the mouth, suggesting that it could play a role in preventing oral cancers. People with oral lesions were given 60 milligrams (100,000 international units) of beta-carotene daily. After 6 months, most of the patients experienced a 50 percent reduction or more in the number of mouth lesions, thus reducing their risk of developing oral cancers.

Medical journals worldwide are filled with studies linking low beta-carotene intake and/or low blood levels of beta-carotene to an increased risk of many different forms of cancer, including cancers of the breast, cervix, lung, stomach, colon and rectum, bladder, mouth, and esophagus. For example, in a recent study, researchers in Buffalo, New York, found that women with breast cancer had lower concentrations of plasma beta-carotene than those who were cancer free. A major study in Latin American countries performed by the National Cancer Institute suggested that a high beta-carotene intake was associated with a 32 percent reduction in cervical cancer.

Heart Disease • Recently, many researchers have begun to believe that atherosclerosis (the clogging of arteries with plaque) may be caused by the oxidation of low-density lipoprotein or "bad" cholesterol. Several studies have shown that beta-carotene can significantly block the oxidation of low-density lipoprotein cholesterol, at least in test tubes. Population studies confirm that people with a high intake of beta-carotene have a lower rate of heart disease than those who don't. For example, ongoing research in the Nurses' Health Study show that by eating even one serving of fruits or vegetables daily, you can reduce your risk of heart attack and stroke. Women in the study who took between 15 and 20 milligrams (25,000 to 33,333 international units) of beta-carotene daily had a 22 percent reduced risk of heart attack and a 40 percent reduced risk of stroke.

Immune Protector • Ultraviolet A (UVA) light from the sun not only promotes wrinkles and skin cancer, but may have harmful effects on the immune system. Researchers at Cornell University and Hoffman-LaRouche tested beta-carotene's ability to protect the immune system from UVA damage. In the study, twenty-four healthy men were put on a low-carotene diet for 28 days. Part of the group took a 30-milligram supplement (50,000 international units) of beta-carotene; the others took a placebo. The whole group was exposed to UVA light several times over the next 2 weeks. Blood tests were then taken to measure the amount of beta-carotene and the ability of the blood to respond to various disease-causing antigens. The results: those on the beta-carotene showed a stronger immune response than those on the placebo.

Another study involved twenty-one patients who tested positive for HIV but did not show any signs of AIDS. These patients were given either 180 milligrams (300,000 international units) of beta-carotene daily or a placebo. Of the seventeen patients who actually completed the 4-week study, the beta-carotene group showed significant increases in several blood factors that help to fight infection. This is not to suggest that beta-carotene is a cure for AIDS; however, it does appear to strengthen the body's immune system.

Cataracts • Several studies have shown that antioxidants in general, and beta-carotene in particular, can protect against the formation of cataracts. According to the Nurses' Health Study, women who eat a diet rich in beta-carotene have a 39 percent lower risk of cataracts than those with a low beta-carotene intake.

PERSONAL ADVICE

Eat a diet rich in dark green leafy vegetables and yellow and orange fruits and vegetables to get the broad-spectrum benefits of beta-carotene.

Bilberry

FACTS

The eyes are one of the most important—and vulnerable—organs, particularly as we age. Reading glasses have become one of the hallmarks of middle age. Later in life, cataracts (growths that cloud the lens of one or both eyes) and macular degeneration (which causes a blur or blind spot in the field of vision) are common occurrences that may be treated surgically, although not always successfully. At any age, exposure to TV and computer screens can lead to eye strain. Bilberry, a common herb, is one of the few known substances that may help preserve precious vision.

Bilberry fruit is grown in Europe and Asia and is similar to the North American blueberry. As with most other herbs, although U.S. scientists have ignored it, serious research on bilberry has been done in Europe, where it is widely used to treat and prevent a number of different disorders.

Bilberry contains biologically active compounds called *anthocyanides*, which may have many positive effects on the body.

THE RIGHT AMOUNT

Bilberry is available in capsule form. Take 1 capsule up to three times daily.

POSSIBLE BENEFITS

Eyes • For centuries, herbal healers have used bilberry to treat eye problems. During World War II, Royal Air Force pilots who munched on sandwiches made of bilberry jam before flying their night missions claimed that the jam improved their night vision. Later, studies confirmed that bilberry does indeed enhance eyesight. In 1964, French researchers found that bilberry improved the adaptation to dark after exposure to bright light. However, the improvement was short-lived; within 24 hours after taking the bilberry, the beneficial effects of this herb had worn off. Later, animal studies revealed that bilberry antho-cyanosides work by accelerating the regeneration of retinol pur-ple (visual purple), a substance that is required for good eyesight, especially at night.

Strengthens Capillaries • Anthrocyanosides have been used as a treatment for capillary fragility (capillaries are extremely narrow blood vessels), a condition that may increase the risk of infection, traumatic injury, and vascular disease. In addition, studies show that bilberry may be a useful tool in preventing vascular disease, which can cause serious circulatory problems in diabetics.

Bioflavonoids

FACTS

Bioflavonoids are a group of about five hundred compounds that provide color to citrus fruits and vegetables. Once regarded as little more than food dye, many of these compounds are now being investigated by the National Cancer Institute for their potential disease preventive properties.

Some bioflavonoids are potent antioxidants. Bioflavonoids are believed to work in conjunction with vitamin C—each may enhance the function of the other. They also work with vitamin C to keep connective tissues healthy. Bioflavonoids are some-times referred to as *vitamin P*, short for capillary permeability factor, because they improve the strength of small blood vessels or capillaries. When the capillary walls are weakened, materials from the blood can penetrate the tissues, which can result in easy bruising or hemorrhaging.

One bioflavonoid, rutin, has been used successfully to treat bleeding gums. Bioflavonoids are used by natural healers to treat allergies and asthma. Synthetic versions of these compounds are used in prescription medications for asthma.

The best food sources of bioflavonoids include the white skin and segment part of citrus fruits, apricots, buckwheat, red and yellow onions, blackberries, cherries, rose hip tea, and apples.

THE RIGHT AMOUNT

There is no recommended daily allowance for bioflavonoids. These compounds are not considered a true vitamin, because no deficiency state has been established. Bioflavonoids are usually available in supplements with vitamin C (the usual combination is 500 milligrams vitamin C to 100 milligrams bioflavonoids). Various bioflavonoids are also sold separately as supplements.

POSSIBLE BENEFITS

Heart Disease • Bioflavonoids appear to offer protection against heart disease. Researchers in Holland evaluated the diets of 805 men aged sixty-five to eighty-four. The group who consumed the highest amounts of bioflavonoids had the lowest rate of heart disease. Researchers speculated that the antioxidant action of bioflavonoids may prevent the oxidizing of low-density lipoprotein cholesterol, which can cause atherosclerosis.

Cancer Fighter • Recent studies show that some bioflavonoids may inhibit the action of carcinogens, thus blocking the initiation of cancerous changes in the cells. In addition, the antioxidant properties of bioflavonoids may also help to prevent cancers caused by oxidative damage. (For example, quercetin, which is found in red and yellow onions, has been shown to inhibit the activity of several carcinogens and tumor promoters.)

Antiviral • Some bioflavonoids have been shown to have antiviral activity, especially in combination with vitamin C. For instance, in one study, a combination of 100 milligrams of vitamin C and 100 milligrams of bioflavonoids dramatically accelerated the healing of cold sores caused by the herpes virus. In test tube studies, quercetin and vitamin C were effective against the coxsackie virus and the common cold.

PERSONAL ADVICE

Bioflavonoids in combination with vitamin D may help to relieve hot flashes associated with menopause. Take 1000 milligrams of bioflavonoids and 400 to 800 international units of vitamin D daily.

Boron

FACTS

Until recently, boron wasn't considered to be of particular importance. There's no recommended daily allowance for boron— like other trace minerals, it is needed by the body in minuscule amounts. However, boron may prove the adage "Good things come in small packages." Although the body only needs a tiny quantity of this mineral, boron may play a big role in helping to prevent osteoporosis and may even help your brain to work better.

Boron is found in most fruits and vegetables; however, dried fruits (e.g., prunes and apricots) are the best source.

THE RIGHT AMOUNT

Take 3 milligrams daily. (Do not exceed 10 milligrams daily.) I recommend boron supplements in the form of sodium borate. Boron works best if taken in a good vitamin and mineral supplement including calcium, magnesium, manganese, and riboflavin.

POSSIBLE BENEFITS

Strong Bones   •   Between 15 and 20 million Americans have osteoporosis, characterized by the thinning or wearing away of bones, which make them more vulnerable to breaks and fractures. Complications from osteoporosis are a leading cause of death among the elderly, especially among women. Recent studies suggest that boron may play an important role in helping the body to retain bone mass. Under the direction of Forrest H. Nielson, Ph.D., supervisory nutritionist, U.S. Department of Agriculture, Agricultural Research Services, researchers tested the effect of boron depletion on twelve postmenopausal women. For 119 days, women were given 2000-calorie diets very low in boron (0.25 milligram). The women were later given the same diet supplemented with 3 milligrams of boron for 48 days. Researchers found that the boron supplement reduced the loss of calcium and magnesium in the urine, both of which are minerals that are needed to help build strong bones. In addition, the boron supplement also dramatically elevated levels of serum estrogen and ionized calcium. This is important because women who develop osteoporosis tend to have low serum estrogen levels and low levels of ionized calcium.

A subsequent study of boron depletion in men and women yielded similar results. In both sexes, boron appears to help the body maintain the essential minerals necessary to prevent bone loss.

Brain Function   •   In a U.S. Department of Agriculture study of boron depletion in men and women over forty-five, subjects on a low-boron diet displayed impaired mental functioning when asked to perform simple tasks such as counting and tapping. Electroencephalograms (a test that measures the electrical activity of the brain) showed that low dietary boron, in the researcher's own words, "depressed mental alertness."

Bromelain

FACTS

Bromelain is an enzyme found in raw pineapple. For several decades, natural food enthusiasts have used bromelain to treat many different ailments, ranging from indigestion to arthritis. Bromelain is beginning to enjoy widespread acceptance among older baby boomers who prefer nature's pharmacy over the synthetic brews found in the conventional pharmacy.

THE RIGHT AMOUNT

Fresh, raw pineapple is a good source of bromelain, although supplements offer a more concentrated form of this enzyme. Bromelain is included in many digestive aid formulas sold at natural food stores. In addition, bromelain tablets are available. Take 1 to 3 daily.

POSSIBLE BENEFITS

Digestive Aid • Bromelain helps to break down protein. As we age, a decrease in hydrochloric acid production can prevent the proper digestion and absorption of protein. A daily bromelain supplement may help to compensate for the loss of HCl.

Anti-inflammatory • Bromelain has anti-inflammatory properties that may help to reduce the discomfort caused by rheumatoid arthritis. There haven't been many clinical studies to confirm this; however, there is a good deal of anecdotal evidence. Due to its anti-inflammatory properties, bromelain is also used by athletes to prevent the soreness that accompanies a strenuous workout. It is also believed to facilitate the healing of sports injuries.

Anti-allergic • Bromelain can also help to alleviate allergic symptoms by mediating the inflammatory response that triggers an allergic attack.

Burdock

FACTS

Called *lappa* in Europe and *gobo* in Japan, the burdock root enjoys worldwide recognition as a mild, nourishing herb that may help to keep the body working well from childhood through old age.

For thousands of years burdock root and leaves have been used to treat rheumatism, gout, and skin disorders, such as psoriasis. The herb has also been used by traditional healers as a cancer treatment (along with other herbs) and is considered to be an excellent digestive aid and liver tonic.

Well-known herbalist Christopher Hobbs includes burdock in his list of *adaptogens,* which he defines as important herbs that can be taken daily without any side effects and help "restore to balance all bodily systems." Herbalist Rosemary Gladstar, author of *Herbal Healing for Women,* prescribes burdock for women in all stages of life.

The Japanese, who have the longest life span of any nationality in the world, frequently eat burdock root. Fresh burdock root is available at many greengrocers, Asian markets, and natural food stores in the United States.

THE RIGHT AMOUNT

Burdock root is available as capsules. Take 1 to 3 daily.

POSSIBLE BENEFITS

Cancer Fighter • Burdock root extracts have been shown to inhibit tumor growth in animal studies.

Liver • Burdock leaves and root are believed to stimulate the production of bile by the liver. Bile is essential for the breakdown of fats.

Fights Infection • Studies show that compounds in burdock have antibacterial and antifungal properties.

PERSONAL ADVICE

According to folklore, a lotion made from the leaves of this root should be massaged into the scalp to prevent hair from falling out.

Butcher's Broom

FACTS

Butcher's broom is one of the most popular anti-aging herbs in Europe, and I predict as word gets out about this herb's healing properties, it will have an equally bright future in the United States.

Butcher's broom contains compounds called *ruscogins*, which are similar in structure to steroids. French studies have shown that butcher's broom is a vasoconstrictor; it strengthens veins and reduces capillary fragility (capillaries are tiny blood vessels).

THE RIGHT AMOUNT

Butcher's broom is available in capsule form. Take 400 milligrams daily. Suppositories and ointments are available to treat hemorrhoidal flareups. Use as directed.

POSSIBLE BENEFITS

Varicose Veins • Blood flows to the heart via a network of arteries and away from the heart via a network of veins. Unlike arteries, which are thick and strong, veins are weaker and less elastic and, therefore, are prone to develop certain problems. When veins become swollen and enlarged, they are called *varicosities*. Varicose veins usually occur in the legs, where blood tends to pool due to poor circulation. Most women over forty develop varicose veins in the legs.

Hemorrhoids—swollen anal veins—are a common ailment

of middle age. Obesity and chronic constipation are risk factors for developing hemorrhoids.

Many European studies show that when used over an extended period of time, butcher's broom can greatly relieve the pain and swelling associated with varicose veins and hemorrhoids. In fact, in Europe, this herb is commonly used for these problems.

Caliciferol (Vitamin D)

FACTS

Calcitrol, or vitamin D, is known as the sunshine vitamin because the ultraviolet B rays of the sun trigger oils of the skin to produce this vitamin. Calcitrol can also be obtained through food. Vitamin D works with calcium and phosphorus to produce strong bones.

The risk of vitamin D deficiency increases with age. Many sunscreens filter out the rays that produce vitamin D. In addition, as we age, our bodies are less able to convert vitamin D into the active hormone that is needed for dietary calcium to become incorporated into bones. If you don't eat a diet rich in vitamin D and if you avoid exposure to the sun (which is wise considering the high rate of skin cancer), you may not be getting enough of this vitamin.

Good food sources of vitamin D are fortified low-fat or no-fat dairy products and fatty fish such as sardines, mackerel, salmon, and tuna.

THE RIGHT AMOUNT

The recommended daily allowance for adults is 400 international units. A recent study suggested that women need 500 international units of vitamin D during the winter to prevent bone loss. Talk to your doctor or natural healer about taking a vitamin D supplement; excessively high doses can be toxic.

POSSIBLE BENEFITS

Osteoporosis • Decreased activity and less exposure to sun can result in wintertime bone loss. According to one study conducted at Tufts University, a vitamin D supplement may help to prevent this loss. In the study, 249 healthy postmenopausal women with a dietary intake of about 100 international units of vitamin D daily were selected to receive a calcium supplement of 800 milligrams per deciliter daily. One-half of the group was given an additional supplement of 400 international units of vitamin D daily. The rest were given a placebo. Researchers then measured the patients' spinal bone mineral density in the summer months and in the winter months. As expected, women in both groups showed an increase in spinal bone mineral density in the summer. However, the women taking the vitamin D supplement showed significantly less bone loss during the winter than those taking the placebo. Based on this study, it would seem wise to take at least 400 international units of vitamin D daily in addition to eating a calcium-rich diet.

Calcium

FACTS

For a lifetime of strong bones, normal blood pressure, and even some protection against cancer, calcium is just what the doctor ordered. Unfortunately, few Americans are filling their prescriptions.

According to a recent U.S. Department of Agriculture survey, most Americans are falling seriously short of this mineral, and the results can be devastating in later life.

Calcium is used for building strong teeth and bones and in maintaining bone strength. It is also important for maintenance of cell membranes, blood clotting, and muscle absorption.

Good sources of calcium are low-fat and nonfat dairy products, kale, broccoli, canned salmon or sardines with bones, and calcium-fortified fruit juice.

THE RIGHT AMOUNT

The recommended daily allowance for adults up to twenty-five is 1200 milligrams, and from twenty-five to fifty, 800 milligrams. Most women and younger men consume less than half the calcium that they need. Postmenopausal women should get 1500 milligrams of calcium daily, but few do.

It may be difficult to obtain all the calcium you need through diet alone. However, recently, several brands of calcium supplements, notably those made from bone meal, dolomite, or oyster shells, tested high in lead. Therefore, I recommend using calcium citrate, which is both safe and effective. Vitamin D helps facilitate calcium absorption.

POSSIBLE BENEFITS

Strong Bones • Twenty-five million Americans—80 percent of them women—have osteoporosis, a condition characterized by low bone mass and increased susceptibility to fractures, primarily in the hip, spine, and wrist. In the United States, osteoporosis is responsible for about 1.3 million fractures per year. Postmenopausal women are particularly vulnerable to this problem; in fact, one-third of all women in their eighties will experience a hip fracture. Complications from osteoporosis are a leading cause of death among elderly women. Recent studies suggest that calcium may play a leading role in helping to reduce bone loss that can lead to osteoporosis.

In a recent French study, more than sixteen hundred postmenopausal women were given 1200 milligrams of calcium and 800 international units of vitamin D daily for 18 months. Another group was given a placebo. The results: a 43 percent reduction in hip fractures among the vitamin-supplemented group. In addition, in the group on calcium and vitamin D, bone density rose 2.7 percent on the hip, whereas density dropped 4.6 percent in the untreated group.

Calcium alone may not be enough to prevent osteoporosis: other studies show that exercise may also play a preventive role as well as postmenopausal estrogen replacement therapy. In fact, for some women, a combination of all three may be their strongest defense against this bone-breaking disease.

Lowers Blood Pressure • High blood pressure, pressure over 140/90, is associated with an increased risk of heart disease and stroke. (The top number, *systolic pressure,* is generated when the heart contracts and pushes blood through the artery. The bottom number, the *diastolic pressure,* is the pressure in the arteries when the heart muscle relaxes between beats.) Several studies have established that calcium supplements can lower blood pressure. A 13-year California study of 6634 men and women showed that people who consumed 1000 milligrams of calcium daily reduced their risk of developing hypertension by 20 percent. Another study of children (the Framingham Children's Study) revealed that the children who ate the most calcium-rich foods had the lowest blood pressures. As we age, blood pressure tends to rise; therefore, adding calcium to your diet may help to prevent developing serious hypertension.

Cancer Protection • Several studies have linked low intake of calcium and vitamin D with an increased risk of colon cancer. For example, a 19-year study of more than 1500 men in Chicago found that an intake of more than 375 milligrams of calcium daily (roughly the amount in one glass of milk) was associated with a 50 percent reduction in the rate of colon cancer as compared to an intake of over 1200 milligrams, which was associated with a 75 percent decrease in colon cancer. Researchers suspect that calcium may bind with fatty acids, thus preventing them from irritating the colon walls. Low intakes of calcium may also increase the rate of excretion of vitamin D, which also appears to play a role in helping to prevent colon cancer. Think of it this way: 2 cups of nonfat milk or calcium-fortified orange juice and two servings of low-fat yogurt may be all that it takes to prevent this potentially lethal cancer.

Capsaicin

FACT

Capsaicin (also known as cayenne), a compound derived from hot chili peppers, gives new meaning to the phrase "Hot 100." Capsaicin is the substance that gives chilies their unique bite. Hot chilies have been used in cooking for thousands of years. Herbal healers have prescribed them for various ailments ranging from asthma to arthritis to even indigestion. (Contrary to popular belief, hot foods do not cause stomach distress in a healthy stomach, although they may irritate ulcers. In fact, chilies actually stimulate the production of saliva and gastric acids, which *aid* digestion.) In recent years, capsaicin has gained the respect of traditional medical practitioners and, ironically, is now considered one of the most important "new" compounds in medicine. Capsaicin has many different affects on the body, and some of them may indeed help to extend life. However, even if capsaicin does not promote longevity, I believe that it can at the very least improve the quality of life for older adults, especially for those in chronic pain.

THE RIGHT AMOUNT

Capsaicin (cayenne) is available in many different forms including capsules, tea, and ointment. Take 1 to 3 capsules daily, or drink 1 cup of tea daily. Capsaicin ointment may be used on the skin for relief of shingles and arthritic pain. Some people may find the ointment irritating, so check with your doctor before using it.

POSSIBLE BENEFITS

Heart Disease • In animal studies, capsaicin has had a favorable effect on blood lipid levels, which can help reduce the risk of heart disease and stroke. According to a 1987 study published in *The Journal of Bioscience*, rats fed a diet high in capsaicin experienced a significant reduction in blood triglycerides and low-density lipoproteins, or "bad" cholesterol. (Triglycerides over 190 milligrams per deciliter for women and over 400 milligrams per deciliter for men are believed to increase the risk of heart attack.)

Pain Relief • When you rub capsaicin cream on your skin, you immediately feel a hot, burning sensation that eventually tapers off. Recently, scientists have learned that capsaicin stimulates certain nerve cells to release a chemical called *substance P*, which sends pain signals throughout the nervous system. Capsaicin quickly depletes the cells of substance P, thus temporarily blocking their ability to transmit any more pain impulses. Capsaicin skin cream is now used topically to treat various ailments, including shingles, a particularly painful rash caused by the reactivation of the chicken pox virus that often strikes older adults. Shingles usually disappears within 3 or 4 weeks; however, in older adults or in people with weakened immune systems, it can linger on in the form of postherpetic neuralgia, a very painful and distressing ailment. A potent form of capsaicin cream (marketed as Zostrix) is one of the few treatments that has offered any relief to the victims of postherpetic neuralgia. In addition, Zostrix has been used quite effectively to treat diabetic neuropathy, a condition characterized by severe foot and ankle pain. Several over-the-counter creams containing capsaicin are also used to treat the pain and stiffness of arthritis. (If you use a cream containing capsaicin, be careful to avoid getting it in your eyes.)

Mood Enhancer • When you bite into a hot chili pepper, you feel a rush of heat that can quite literally bring tears to your eyes. The body responds to this "pain" by releasing *endorphins,* chemicals in the brain that have a pain-relieving effect similar to morphine. Capsaicin may be nature's way of helping you to beat the blues.

PERSONAL ADVICE

Cayenne tea can have a mild, stimulating effect. When you're feeling down, have a cup for a quick pick-me-up.

L-Carnitine

FACTS

If you're at risk of developing coronary artery disease (the number one killer in the United States of both men and women), here's a potential life extender that you should know about. L-Carnitine is a nonprotein amino acid that is found in heart and skeletal muscle. Its primary job is to carry activated fatty acids across the mitochondria—the so-called powerhouse of the cell—providing heart and skeletal cells with energy.

L-Carnitine is widely used in Japan as a treatment for heart disease and is growing in popularity in the United States. Enthusiasts claim that L-Carnitine can protect against heart disease and can improve physical stamina and endurance during exercise.

Severe L-Carnitine deficiency is fairly rare and is associated with muscle weakness and cramps after exercise. People with kidney disease, severe infection, liver disease, and other medical problems may develop L-Carnitine deficiency. Some researchers believe that subtle forms of L-Carnitine deficiency, which may go unnoticed, may increase the risk of having a heart attack.

Red meat—beef and lamb—and dairy products are the best natural sources of L-Carnitine. Unfortunately, these foods are also high in saturated fat, which can promote heart disease. Therefore, an L-Carnitine supplement may be preferable to loading up on meat.

THE RIGHT AMOUNT

There is no recommended daily allowance for L-Carnitine. The average American consumes between 100 and 300 milligrams of this amino acid daily. L-Carnitine is available in capsule form at natural food stores. Take two 500-milligram capsules daily. In rare cases, people taking over 1 gram of carnitine per day may develop a fishy odor, which is caused by the breakdown of carnitine by intestinal bacteria. The odor usually disappears when the dose is cut back; however, if it is troublesome, you may want to discontinue use.

Caution: There are two kinds of carnitine: L-carnitine **and** D-carnitine. **Some studies suggest that** D-carnitine **may be toxic, therefore, stick to products containing only** L-carnitine. **If you have a heart condition, do not take this or any other supplement without first consulting with your physician. In high doses (over 3 grams per day),** L-carnitine **may cause cramps or diarrhea.**

POSSIBLE BENEFITS

Heart Disease • Ischemia is the reduction in the oxygen supply to the heart usually caused by the narrowing of a coronary artery, often due to atherosclerotic deposits or an arterial spasm. Several studies show that ischemia can result in a reduction in carnitine in heart muscle. L-Carnitine supplements appear to raise carnitine levels in heart patients and increase their endurance. In one study involving eighteen patients with coronary artery disease, exercise sessions were performed 2 weeks apart. Prior to exercise, one group of patients received carnitine, and the other received a placebo. Those on carnitine maintained lower blood pressure and were able to exercise longer and harder prior to experiencing angina or chest pain (a sign of ischemia). Other studies of heart patients have yielded similar results. We don't know for sure whether L-Carnitine supplements can actually prevent ischemia, but these studies suggest that it might.

In another study, twenty-six patients with high blood lipid levels were treated with 3 grams of oral L-Carnitine per day. The result: a dramatic decline in total serum cholesterol and serum triglyceride. (Cholesterol levels over 200 milligrams per deciliter may increase your risk of having a heart attack. Triglyceride levels over 400 for men, and 190 for women are believed to increase the risk of heart disease.) In other studies, L-Carnitine has been shown to raise high-density lipoproteins, or "good" cholesterol.

Improves Workout • I have heard anecdotal evidence that L-Carnitine can improve stamina and strength during a workout; however, there is no scientific evidence.

Alzheimer's Disease • The brain tissue of mammals is a rich source of carnitine. Some studies suggest that L-Carnitine may be effective in slowing down the progression of Alzheimer's disease. Several European studies have reported that a daily supplement of L-Carnitine (about 2 grams daily) can slow the mental deterioration typical of this disease. (Dietary intakes of L-Carnitine average 100 to 300 milligrams daily in the United States.) However, U.S. researchers did not report good results from a major trial testing L-Carnitine on Alzheimer's patients.

Centella (Gotu Kola)

FACTS

Although most people can maintain good health throughout their lifetime, there are times when an accident or illness may result in prolonged bed rest or reduced activity. Centella (also called gotu kola) can help you get back on your feet faster by preventing dangerous complications that can result during an extended period of inactivity.

THE RIGHT AMOUNT

Centella is available as capsules or extract. Take 1 capsule up to three times daily. Mix 5 to 10 drops of extract in a cup of liquid. Take up to three times daily.

Caution: Do not use this herb during pregnancy. People with an overactive thyroid should avoid this herb.

POSSIBLE BENEFITS

Circulatory Disorders • Patients confined to bed can develop venous insufficiency, a condition that seriously impairs the flow of blood throughout the body, especially in the feet and legs. In some cases, the veins may become inflamed, resulting in phlebitis, a painful and potentially serious condition. Compounds in centella have been shown to strengthen and tone veins and capillaries and may help prevent circulatory problems. In addition, studies show that centella has been used successfully to treat patients suffering from problems related to venous insufficiency.

Wound Healing • Used externally or taken internally, centella can accelerate the healing of wounds, skin ulcers, and other sores.

PERSONAL ADVICE

According to herbalist Christopher Hobbs, legend has it that if you eat a leaf of centella each day, your life span will be extended one thousand years.

Choline

FACTS

Thousands of years ago, Chinese healers recommended foods such as eggs and meat for mental alertness and foods such as fruits and grains for a more relaxed state. Until recently, modern psychiatry dismissed such notions as pure hokum, but we now know that the chemicals in foods can indeed have a profound effect on our thought processes and mental well-being.

For example, egg yolks contain a compound called *phosphatidylcholine*, which is a major source of choline in the body.

Recent studies suggest that choline may prove to be a memory tonic.

The brain consists of millions of tiny neurons or cells that are connected by long tendrils called *axons*. The cells "talk" to each other via chemicals called *neurotransmitters*. The brain uses choline to make acetylcholine, a neurotransmitter that plays a role in memory function.

Other good food sources of choline include soybeans, cabbage, peanuts, and cauliflower.

THE RIGHT AMOUNT

Choline is available in tablet and liquid form at natural food stores. Take 1000 milligrams daily.

POSSIBLE BENEFITS

Memory Booster • Some researchers believe that as we age, we begin to produce less acetylcholine or the acetylcholine that is produced is less efficient, which is why many older people become forgetful. There is some evidence that choline deficiency may result in memory loss. Alzheimer's patients have lower levels of choline than normal. However, attempts to reverse the condition with choline supplements have so far been ineffective. Some researchers believe, however, that choline supplementation may slow down memory loss.

In another study, a drug that interferes with acetylcholine was given to college students. The students began to show signs of forgetfulness similar to those seen among the elderly. In fact, many common drugs, including antihistamines, antidepressants, and antispasmodics, may block acetylcholine and can cause short-term memory loss. Older people in particular are especially vulnerable to drug-induced memory loss and are quick to assume that lapses in memory are a natural part of the aging process. Very often, memory is restored when the drugs are stopped.

Chromium

FACTS

When you were a kid, nobody ever told you, "Take your chromium or no dessert!" Now that you're *not* a kid anymore, I'd like to remind you, "Take your chromium." As we age, we need this mineral more than ever.

Chromium is a trace mineral that works with insulin to help the body utilize sugar and metabolize fat. Recent studies suggest that chromium protects against heart disease and diabetes and may even help to firm up flabby muscles. What's even more exciting is the fact that a preliminary study hints that chromium may improve longevity.

Chromium is found in broccoli, whole wheat English muffins, brewer's yeast, meat, cheese, and shellfish.

THE RIGHT AMOUNT

There is no recommended daily allowance for chromium. In 1980, the National Research Council, National Academy of Sciences, recommended 50 to 200 micrograms of chromium daily. Richard Anderson, Ph.D., of the U.S. Department of Agriculture's Human Nutrition Research Center—a leading authority in chromium—says that people need at least 50 micrograms daily of chromium. However, he concedes that most Americans fall short of this amount. Studies show that serum chromium levels decrease with age, which means that adults over fifty are often short on chromium.

I recommend taking a minimum of 200 micrograms of chromium daily.

POSSIBLE BENEFITS

Improves Glucose Tolerance • Insulin helps the body to metabolize or break down glucose, or blood sugar, in a form that can be utilized by cells for energy. Animal studies show that chromium helps regulate the release of insulin by acting on insulin-producing cells or beta cells. Beta cells in the pancreas manufacture and store insulin until a rising blood sugar level signals to them to release it. In a U.S. Department of Agriculture study, one group of laboratory rats was fed a chromium-rich diet; the other was fed a chromium-deficient diet. Each group of rats was given a glucose solution to stimulate insulin. The rats fed the chromium-deficient diet secreted up to 50 percent less insulin during the test than the rats given the chromium-sufficient diet. Based on this study, it appears as if chromium directly stimulates the production of insulin as the body needs it.

Human studies show that chromium supplements can normalize blood sugar levels in half the people with high blood sugar.

As people age, there is a tendency to develop type II diabetes mellitus, a condition characterized by high blood glucose levels often caused by the body's failure to produce enough insulin. Researchers are hopeful that chromium may help to perk up insulin production in older adults, thus reducing the risk of developing this form of diabetes.

Lowers Blood Lipids • Several studies have shown that chromium can cut serum cholesterol levels and triglycerides, another form of blood lipid that may help to promote heart disease. In a study published in *The Western Journal of Medicine*, twenty-eight volunteers with elevated cholesterol (220 to 320 milligrams per deciliter) were given either 200 micrograms of chromium picolinate supplement or a placebo. After a 6-week period, those on the chromium showed an average 7 percent drop in cholesterol, thus reducing their risk of heart disease by 14 percent. Low-density lipoprotein, or "bad" cholesterol, levels dipped by more than 10 percent.

Muscle Builder • Chromium picolinate supplements are being promoted as a new and safe way to build muscle. Several studies have shown that supplements of chromium picolinate can increase muscle mass. However, it only works for people who exercise regularly. Therefore, if you want to firm up the flab, take a chromium supplement along with a sensible exercise regime. Sorry, couch potatoes, simply popping a chromium pill without exercise is not effective. (As we went to press, a recent study suggested that this popular form of chromium, chromium picolinate, may cause chromosomal damage on animal cells in high doses. We do not know whether this is significant for humans or not.)

Longevity • I've saved the best for last. A researcher at Bemidji State University in Minnesota fed chromium picolinate and two other chromium supplements to a small group of laboratory rats. The results: the rats on the chromium picolinate lived an average of 1 year longer than the rats on the other form of chromium. The chromium picolinate increased the average life span of the rats by one-third. Although we don't know whether chromium will help humans live longer, we do know that chromium can help prevent heart disease and diabetes, which can cut life short.

Cinnamon

FACTS

Cinnamon has been a highly prized spice since ancient times and is used in many different cuisines. However, modern scientists are finding some new uses for this venerable spice. Recently, researchers have discovered that cinnamon (and a handful of other spices) may help control blood sugar levels by increasing the efficiency of insulin.

THE RIGHT AMOUNT

Use this spice freely on cereal, fruit, yogurt, and even toast. I make it a point to eat about 1 teaspoon of cinnamon daily.

POSSIBLE BENEFITS

Diabetes • About one in four Americans have a genetic tendency to develop *diabetes*, a condition characterized by the inability of the body to metabolize and use foods properly. As a result, diabetics develop excessive amounts of blood sugar that is not utilized and is secreted into urine. In many cases, the diabetic does not produce enough *insulin*, the hormone that helps to regulate blood sugar. Insulin is produced by beta cells in the pancreas, and over time, these beta cells can wear out. If untreated, diabetes can lead to severe complications including heart disease. Most cases of diabetes occur later in life; in fact, a sixty-five-year-old is sixty times more likely to develop diabetes than someone under twenty. Even if you have a tendency to develop diabetes, it is not inevitable that you will. Some physicians believe that the condition can be delayed or even avoided through proper diet. People who are overweight, especially women, are at much higher risk of developing diabetes than normal-weight people. A high-fat, high-calorie diet may overwhelm the beta cells, hastening the onset of diabetes. However, some foods and spices appear to help keep blood sugar levels under control. In recent test tube studies, cinnamon appeared to significantly increase the ability of insulin to metabolize glucose.

Citrus

FACTS

Will eating citrus fruit make you live longer? The National Cancer Institute (NCI) is banking on it. The NCI is spending millions of dollars to study compounds found in oranges, grapefruit, lemons, and limes for their potential cancer-fighting properties.

Citrus fruits contain a virtual drug store of phytochemicals that may help to ward off disease. However, they are best known for being an excellent source of vitamin C, a potent antioxidant and enemy of the common cold. In addition, citrus fruits offer other important minerals including potassium, which controls blood pressure, and a fair amount of fiber, which is good for most everything.

THE RIGHT AMOUNT

Make one of your "five a day" a citrus fruit.

POSSIBLE BENEFITS

Cancer Fighter • The NCI is investigating *limonene*, a citrus oil that has been shown to shrink mammary tumors in rats and, even better, prevented the growth of new tumors. Given the fact that breast cancer is a virtual epidemic in the United States, limonene may prove to be of great importance.

Citrus also contains compounds called *bioflavonoids* (also known as vitamin P), which provide the yellow and orange color of these fruits and maybe much, much more. Some bioflavonoids are antioxidants that help prevent damage to cells inflicted by free radicals. Others help to prevent the spread of malignant cells throughout the body. Researchers hope that one day a form of bioflavonoids may be used to treat various forms of cancer.

In addition, citrus contains *terpenes*, compounds that help produce enzymes that deactivate carcinogens (and also limit the production of cholesterol), which may also prove to be a useful tool in the fight against cancer.

Heart Disease • Most heart attacks and strokes are caused by tiny blood clots that form in arteries that are already narrowed by atherosclerotic lesions. Citrus contains *coumarins*, natural blood thinners that may help prevent the formation of dangerous clots.

Pectin, a compound found in the pulpy membranes that separate individual sections in grapefruits and oranges, can lower blood cholesterol levels, thus reducing the risk of heart attack and stroke. Grapefruit pectin is the most effective. In a recent study at the University of Florida College of Medicine, people with high cholesterol levels were given grapefruit pectin (in a powdered form) daily. Within 16 weeks, the group's cholesterol dropped on average 7.6 percent; low-density lipoproteins, or "bad" cholesterol, were cut by 10 percent. Although the powdered form of grapefruit may be more potent than the natural pectin, researchers believe that whole grapefruit can also lower cholesterol, although perhaps not as much. However, since most people only eat the grapefruit sections and not the membrane containing the pectin, they miss out on the cholesterol-lowering benefit.

Club Moss

FACTS

For centuries, Chinese healers have routinely prescribed a tea brewed from an oriental club moss (*Huperzia serrata*) to reverse memory loss in older people. Western scientists, who tended to dismiss all folk medicine, have tried to no avail to concoct their own drug to reinvigorate people's memories. In 1986, skepticism gave way to hope when researchers at the Shanghai Institute of Materia Medica reported that they had isolated natural compounds in club moss called *huperzine A* and *huperzine B*, which, according to animal tests, helped to improve learning, memory retrieval, and memory retention. (Huperzine A appeared to be the more effective.)

What Western scientists found most intriguing about huperzine was that it raised acetylcholine levels by inhibiting acetylcholinesterase, an enzyme that breaks down acetylcholine. Acetylcholine is a chemical found in the brain that is directly involved in memory and awareness. People with Alzheimer's disease, a life-threatening disorder characterized by severe memory loss and dementia, have lower than normal levels of acetylcholine. Because there is no treatment or cure for

Alzheimer's, any compound that can raise acetylcholine levels is considered a potential weapon against this debilitating disease. Researchers at the Mayo Clinic in Jacksonville, Florida, have been studying huperzine as a potential drug for Alzheimer's. They have recently licensed the use of huperzine A to a pharmaceutical company that is seeking the Food and Drug Administration's permission to test the drug on humans.

THE RIGHT AMOUNT

Drink 1 or 2 cups of brewed club moss tea daily. There are several different types of club moss; be sure that the tea is *Huperzia serrata* and not some other species of club moss. (The species of club moss native to the United States has not yet been studied, so there is no way of knowing whether it would be effective.) Depending on where you live, getting true club moss may be a bit of a challenge; however, it should be available at major herb stores around the country. If you live in an area with a large Chinese population, check out some of the local herb shops.

POSSIBLE BENEFITS

Memory Enhancer • Several animal studies confirm huperzine A's positive effect on memory. In one study, laboratory mice were taught how to run through an electric grid without getting a shock. After the training, the mice were given either an electric shock or a drug to induce amnesia. One group of mice was given huperzine immediately after the amnesia treatment, the other group was not. Twenty-four hours later, the mice were placed back on the electric grid to see how much they retained from their earlier training. The mice given huperzine performed significantly better than the untreated mice. Will huperzine work as well on humans? There are some promising signs that it will. For example, Chinese studies have shown that huperzine can help to improve memory function in stroke victims. More studies are needed before we know for sure whether huperzine will offer relief from Alzheimer's disease and whether it really is a potent memory tonic. However, in the meantime, it can't hurt to include a cup or two of club moss tea in your daily diet.

Cobalamin (Vitamin B_{12})

FACTS

Cobalamin, also known as vitamin B_{12}, plays many important roles in the body. It aids in the production of red blood cells, is essential for the normal functioning of the nervous system, and also helps to metabolize protein and fat. Most recently, B_{12} has been touted as the "brain vitamin," because a lack of this important vitamin can severely hamper mental agility in people of all ages. B_{12} deficiency is quite common among the elderly population. In fact, as many as 10 percent of people over sixty may have low blood levels of this vitamin, and the results can be devastating.

B_{12} is found in meat, fish, eggs, and dairy products.

THE RIGHT AMOUNT

The recommended daily allowance for B_{12} is 2 micrograms for men and women. B_{12} is available as capsules, tablets, a nasal gel, and a sublingual form that dissolves under the tongue.

POSSIBLE BENEFITS

Brain Booster • According to a recent study performed at the University Hospital of Maastricht in the Netherlands, otherwise healthy people with low blood levels of B_{12} did not perform as well on mental tests as people with higher blood levels of this vitamin, regardless of age.

Neurologic Symptoms in Older Adults • Vitamin B_{12} deficiency can cause severe neurologic and psychological symptoms in older people, ranging from numbness or tingling in the arms or legs (peripheral neuropathy) to balance problems, to confusion and even dementia. If caught in time, many but not all of these problems can be reversed with B_{12} supplements. Unfortunately, many people are likely to dismiss confusion or erratic behavior in the elderly as part of the natural aging process and may not look for other causes. However, several studies show that B_{12} deficiency is extremely widespread among people over sixty. In fact, according to a recent study of one hundred people between ages sixty-five and ninety-three performed at New York Medical College, more than twenty-one had *low* B_{12} levels (of which two had peripheral neuropathy) and sixteen had *very low* levels (of which three had peripheral neuropathy and one suffered from mental deterioration).

Why is B_{12} deficiency so common among older adults? As people age, they are prone to develop a condition called *atrophic gastritis*, characterized by less gastric acid and an increased amount of bacteria in the upper small intestine and stomach. The combination of a low level of gastric acid and the presence of bacteria is believed to hamper the ability of the body to utilize the B_{12} in food. Antibiotics may be prescribed to reduce the level of bacteria, which may help increase the level of B_{12} derived from food. However, B_{12} supplements may be better absorbed than B_{12} bound to food.

If an older person shows signs of neurologic or psychological disturbances and other physical causes have been ruled out, he or she should be checked for B_{12} deficiency. In fact, some researchers now believe that every adult over sixty-five should be checked for B_{12} deficiency since the long-term consequences can be devastating.

PERSONAL ADVICE

I personally recommend the nasal gel or sublingual form, which bypasses the stomach and is directly absorbed into the bloodstream.

Coenzyme Q_{10}

FACTS

An *enzyme* is a protein found in living cells that brings about chemical changes. A coenzyme works with an enzyme to produce a particular reaction. Coenzyme Q_{10} is found in every cell in the body and is essential in facilitating the process that provides cells with energy. As we age, levels of cozenzyme Q_{10} begin to fall. However, exercise can raise levels of coenzyme Q_{10}.

Coenzyme Q_{10} can be synthesized by the body or obtained from food. Deficiency states can occur, particularly among the elderly.

Since 1974, coenzyme Q_{10} has been used successfully to treat heart disease in Japan—6 million Japanese take it annually. Recent studies suggest that coenzyme Q_{10} may play a vital role in thwarting the aging process. It can also increase your energy level, especially in people who do not exercise.

THE RIGHT AMOUNT

Coenzyme Q_{10} is available as capsules. Take 30 milligrams daily.

POSSIBLE BENEFITS

Heart Disease   •   Several studies have shown that coenzyme Q_{10} can increase stamina and reduce angina in heart patients. In one Japanese study, researchers selected ten men and two women with chronic unstable angina (chest pain) between the ages of forty-five and sixty-six. The 12-week study was divided into three phases. In phase 1, patients were given a placebo. In phase 2, half the patients were given a placebo, and the others were given 150 milligrams of coenzyme Q_{10} daily (50 milligrams three times a day). In phase 3, the group on the placebo was given coenzyme Q_{10}, and the group that had been given coenzyme Q_{10} was now given a placebo. During each phase, exercise tests were performed by patients on a treadmill. Patients on the coenzyme Q_{10} had fewer attacks of angina and were able to exercise longer than those not on the medication. In addition, those on the coenzyme Q_{10} required fewer nitroglycerin tablets to relieve the pain of angina than those on the placebo.

In Japan, coenzyme Q_{10} is used to treat congestive heart failure. It works by increasing the strength of the heart muscle.

Studies have shown that coenzyme Q_{10} may lower blood pressure.

Antioxidant • Animal studies have shown that coenzyme Q_{10} inhibits *lipid peroxidation,* a process that promotes the formation of *free radicals,* unstable oxygen molecules that can cause damage and malignant changes in cells. Free radicals may contribute to heart disease, premature aging, and even cancer. Antioxidants such as coenzyme Q_{10} may prevent cells from being damaged by free radicals.

PERSONAL ADVICE

Coenzyme Q_{10} is very effective in preventing toxicity from a large number of drugs used to treat cancer, high blood pressure, and other diseases.

Cranberry

FACTS

Urinary tract infections (UTIs), characterized by painful urination, blood or pus in the urine, fever, low back pain, or cramps, are more common among older men and women. In men, enlargement of the prostate gland, a common condition affecting nearly half of all men over fifty, can promote UTIs. Postmenopausal women in particular suffer more UTIs than younger women due to vaginal dryness caused by lower estrogen levels.

Once an infection has taken hold, it must be properly treated with medication, and sometimes, several drugs must be used before the infection is gone. However, studies have shown that cranberry juice can help prevent these annoying and painful infections from occurring in the first place.

THE RIGHT AMOUNT

Drink 1 to 2 glasses of cranberry juice daily. Cranberry concentrate is available in capsule form at natural food stores. Take 2 to 6 capsules daily.

POSSIBLE BENEFITS

Prevent UTIs • UTIs are caused by *Escherichia coli* bacterium, which tends to adhere to the walls of the urinary tract. Recently, researchers at Alliance City Hospital in Ohio discovered that cranberry juice prevented *Escherichia coli* from sticking to the endothelial cells of the urinary tract; thus, the potentially dangerous bacterium was flushed out in the urine.

Cruciferous Vegetables

FACTS

Population studies of dietary habits—so-called epidemiological studies—have shown that people who eat a diet high in cruciferous vegetables (e.g., cabbage, broccoli, brussels sprouts, kale, and cauliflower) have lower rates of cancer than people who don't. Because of its possible role in fighting cancer, researchers at the National Cancer Institute have begun investigating the cruciferous family to isolate its potential cancer-fighting properties.

THE RIGHT AMOUNT

I recommend at least two servings (1 cup) of these vegetables daily.

POSSIBLE BENEFITS

Cancer Fighter   •   Researchers at the Institute for Hormone Research in New York have found that *indoles,* a group of phytochemicals in cruciferous vegetables, may be a powerful weapon against cancer. Indoles appear to alter the biological pathway that converts certain estrogens into more potent forms that can trigger the growth of tumors in estrogen-sensitive sites, such as the breast. Women with breast cancer tend to have higher blood estrogen levels than normal, and any substance that controls the amount of estrogen circulating in the bloodstream may have a protective effect against certain forms of breast cancer.

Researchers at Johns Hopkins School of Medicine in Baltimore recently found what may be an even more vigorous cancer fighter in cruciferous vegetables: *sulforaphane.* Sulforaphane stimulates the action of protective enzymes that help the body fight against tumor growth. (See Sulforaphane, p. 150.) In fact, one researcher said that sulforaphane may be one of the most potent protective agents against cancer discovered to date!

Antioxidant Boost   •   Cruciferous vegetables are excellent sources of beta-carotene, vitamin C, selenium, and vitamin E. Antioxidants may help to prevent the cellular damage caused by free radicals, which may be responsible for many different forms of cancer and heart disease.

Fiber Boost   •   Cruciferous vegetables are an excellent source of fiber, which helps to prevent constipation and digestive diseases, such as diverticulosis, but also may help to prevent cancer of the colon, breast, lung, and cervix.

Dandelion

FACTS

To most suburbanites, dandelions are just troublesome weeds. But to practitioners of herbal medicine, they are a veritable gold mine. Herbalists have long used dandelions to treat liver ailments and digestive disorders. Like so many other herbs these days, dandelions are being rediscovered by men and women who are determined to maintain a lifetime of good health.

Dandelion is an excellent source of beta-carotene and lutein, two members of the carotenoid family that may protect against certain forms of cancer.

THE RIGHT AMOUNT

Dandelions can be eaten fresh in salads. Dandelion tea and capsules are available at natural food stores. Drink 1 cup of tea daily or take 1 to 3 capsules daily. Dandelion is included in many herbal formulas designed to promote good digestion and improve liver function.

POSSIBLE BENEFITS

Liver • The liver weighs a mere 3 to 4 pounds, but it is worth its weight in gold several times over. The liver performs many vital jobs in the body including the detoxification of poisons and impurities that may enter the bloodstream; the production of sex hormones, proteins, and enzymes; and the breakdown of fat. Animal studies show that dandelion extract can stimulate the production of bile by the liver, which is essential for the metabolism of fat. Herbalists believe that dandelion is an overall tonic for the liver, generally improving the liver's ability to function.

Digestive Aid • Dandelion, like other "bitters," can help treat digestive problems, such as gas and bloating. This herb can also help to prevent constipation.

Menopause • Dandelion, which is rich in plant estrogens, is often prescribed to relieve some of the discomfort of menopause caused by a sharp dip in estrogen levels. Dandelion has a mild diuretic effect, which can help eliminate menopausal water retention. However, unlike other diuretics, it is rich in potassium and does not sap the body of this vital mineral.

Dong Quai

FACTS

Known in the West as dong quai and in the Far East as tang keui, this member of the angelica family is a highly esteemed anti-aging herb. According to Ron Teeguarden, author of *Chinese Tonic Herbs*, dong quai is the "ultimate woman's tonic herb." It is widely used throughout Asia to help ease the symptoms of menopause.

In younger women, dong quai is used to regulate menstrual disorders.

THE RIGHT AMOUNT

Dong quai is available in tablet or capsule form and is included in many "change of life" supplements sold at natural food stores. Take 2 tablets or capsules twice daily.

POSSIBLE BENEFITS

Menopause • Chinese healers consider dong quai to be a hormone regulator that maintains hormones within normal levels. Dong quai contains hormonelike compounds that may relieve hot flashes, vaginal dryness, and other symptoms of menopause. It is also rich in vitamin E, which may also explain why women may find it useful for menopause. Dong quai has a mild sedative effect, which can help relieve stress.

Heart Disease   •   Studies show that this herb can lower blood pressure in both men and women and slow down the pulse rate.

Anemia   •   Chinese women use dong quai as a "blood builder." Dong quai is a rich source of iron and may help to prevent iron deficiency anemia.

Diabetes   •   Dong quai has been shown to regulate blood sugar, thus helping to prevent high concentrations of glucose or blood sugar that can lead to diabetes.

PERSONAL ADVICE

Next time you're eating at a Cantonese Chinese restaurant, try ordering the dong quai duck.

Echinacea

FACTS

Echinacea is living proof that the more things change, the more they stay the same. Native Americans first used this beautiful purple cornflower as a remedy for toothaches, sore throats, and even snake bites. European settlers brought echinacea back to Europe, where it quickly became a popular herbal remedy. Around the turn of the century, scientists who had studied the effect of echinacea on blood cultures recognized that this herb could boost the immune system by stimulating the production of white blood cells. Physicians as well as herbalists used echinacea to treat infection and cancer. Once antibiotics were discovered, interest in herbs such as echinacea waned. However, as interest in preventive medicine increased in the 1980s, researchers began to look for ways to keep people healthy. Anything that could bolster the immune system attracted great attention, and interest in echinacea was revived. Today, as we approach the twenty-first century, echinacea is now being touted as a hot "new" immunostimulant.

THE RIGHT AMOUNT

Echinacea is available in capsule and extract forms at most natural food stores and herb shops. (Some preparations are made from the roots of the *Echinacea angustifolia* plant; others are made from the roots or leaves of *Echinacea purpurea*.) Either form of echinacea may be included in herbal preparations designed to boost the immune system.

I find that the capsules are the easiest. Take 1 capsule three times daily. If you prefer to use extract, mix 15 to 30 drops in liquid every 3 hours up to three times daily. Many of the active compounds in echinacea can be destroyed during processing. Freeze-drying is the most effective way to preserve this herb's healing properties.

POSSIBLE BENEFITS

Antiviral • Several studies have shown that echinacea prevents the formation of an enzyme called *hyaluronidase*, which destroys a natural barrier between healthy tissue and unwanted pathogenic organisms. Thus, echinacea helps cells maintain their natural line of defense against bacteria and viruses.

Several studies have shown that echinacea may be an effective treatment against colds, ear infections, and flu. A recent German study of 180 patients between the ages of eighteen and sixty showed that echinacea extract (four droppers daily) were significant in relieving the symptoms and duration of flulike infections. (There's no reason to believe that capsules would not work as well.) Other European studies have shown that echinacea is useful in the treatment of ear infections in children.

In 1978, a study of echinacea in *Planta Medica* showed that a root extract destroyed both herpes and influenza virus.

Cancer Fighter • Several animal studies show that echinacea can inhibit the growth of certain types of tumors, probably by stimulating the production of key lymphocytes, which in turn accelerate the body's own defenses. Echinacea has also been used to restore normal immune function in patients receiving chemotherapy.

Antifungal • At least one study has shown that echinacea (taken orally and applied vaginally in cream form) may be an effective treatment against yeast infection (*Candida albicans*), a particularly persistent infection. Even better, this treatment appears to help prevent the infection from recurring.

Ellagic Acid

FACTS

Ellagic acid, a polyphenolic compound found in fruit, is attracting a great deal of attention among cancer researchers because it appears to be a potent cancer fighter.

Strawberries, grapes, and cherries are a good source of ellagic acid.

THE RIGHT AMOUNT

There is no recommended daily allowance for ellagic acid. As of yet, there is not enough information to recommend a specific amount of ellagic acid; however, I advise people to eat at least one serving daily of a fruit with this substance (one serving = ½ cup of fruit).

As of this writing, ellagic acid is not available in supplement form. Even if it were, I generally advise people to try to get their phytochemicals from food whenever possible.

POSSIBLE BENEFITS

Cancer Fighter • Animal studies show that ellagic acid counteracts synthetic and naturally occurring carcinogens, thus preventing healthy cells form turning cancerous. Ellagic acid is also an antioxidant, which may block the destructive effects of free radicals.

Ellagic acid's ability to counteract carcinogens is very promising. For example, in one Japanese study, laboratory rats were fed a diet high in various polyphenol compounds. One group was given ellagic acid exclusively. The rats were later exposed to a potent carcinogen to induce tongue cancer. All of the rats on the various polyphenolic compounds had a reduced incidence of cancer; however, those on the ellagic acid remained entirely cancer free. The researchers speculated that ellagic acid (and other polyphenols) may help to prevent cancer in other tissues, including the skin, lung, liver, and esophagus.

In another study, researchers tested the effect of ellagic acid on a nicotine-derived carcinogen found in cigarette smoke. The study revealed that the ellagic acid (and other polyphenols) blocked the carcinogenic effect of the nicotine compound on animal cells.

More research needs to be done to determine if ellagic acid will work in a similar way on humans. However, until the results are in, eating foods rich in ellagic acid can't hurt, and it just might help.

Fenugreek

FACTS

Fenugreek is an herb that is used as a spice to flavor curry and chutney. Since ancient times, it has been valued for its medicinal properties. Fenugreek is reputed to be an aphrodisiac. It has been used to treat impotence in men and discomfort associated with menopause in women. Modern scientists believe that fenugreek may play a role in helping to prevent or postpone adult-onset diabetes.

THE RIGHT AMOUNT

Fenugreek tea is available at natural food stores. It is also available in capsule form. Drink 1 to 2 cups daily. Take 1 capsule up to three times daily. It is also included in many herbal formulas for women.

Caution: Do not use fenugreek during pregnancy.

POSSIBLE BENEFITS

Menopause • Fenugreek contains steroidal saponins, which are similar to sex hormones produced by the body and, therefore, may play a role in regulating hormone levels. In fact, herbal healers recommend fenugreek for hot flashes and depression associated with menopause.

Diabetes • According to U.S. Department of Agriculture researcher James A. Duke, Ph.D., fenugreek (along with a handful of other herbs and spices) may help slow the onset of adult diabetes. Fenugreek seeds contain at least six different compounds that can help control blood sugar levels, thus preventing a sugar surge that may create problems for many older people who may not produce enough insulin or may be insulin resistant.

Fiber

FACTS

There's one thing that advocates for alternative medicine and mainstream groups like the American Medical Association can agree on: Americans should eat more fiber.

Fiber is a catchall phrase for the nonnutritive food substances found in plants that are not digested or absorbed by the body—so-called roughage. Although there is compelling evidence that a diet high in fiber may help to ward off a number of deadly diseases, the American diet is woefully low in fiber. In fact, the average American consumes about 10 grams of fiber daily, less than half of the 30 grams of fiber recommended by most doctors and medical researchers.

There are two types of fiber: soluble and insoluble.

Soluble fiber, which includes pectin and plant gums, binds with bile in the intestine and is excreted in the feces. Scientists believe that the liver compensates for the loss of bile by producing more bile salts in which cholesterol is a necessary ingredient. By reducing the amount of cholesterol circulating in the blood, soluble fiber helps to lower blood cholesterol levels.

Insoluble fiber contains compounds called *cellulose* and *hemocelluloses,* which absorb water and can improve the functioning of the large bowel. Insoluble fiber softens and bulks waste to help move it more quickly through the colon, thus helping to prevent constipation and reducing exposure to pesticides or naturally occurring carcinogens in food.

Good sources of soluble fiber include apples, oat bran, broccoli, carrots, dried peas and beans, potatoes, strawberries, and other fruits and vegetables.

Good sources of insoluble fiber include celery, leafy green vegetables, whole grains, kidney and pinto beans, apples, and other fruits and vegetables.

THE RIGHT AMOUNT

I recommend 30 to 35 grams of fiber daily. In order to achieve this goal, you must be diligent about consuming daily at least five servings of fruits and vegetables daily (½ cup or one medium size fruit = one serving) and roughly six servings of whole grains (one piece of whole grain bread or ½ cup of whole grain cereal = one serving).

Caution: If you're adding fiber to your diet, go slow! Introduce it gradually. If you gobble up too much fiber too quickly, you may develop gas and cramps. Drinking 6 to 8 glasses of water daily will help relieve gas.

If you have any rectal bleeding or blood in your stool, contact your doctor immediately.

POSSIBLE BENEFITS

Cancer Fighter • In 1970, British physician Dr. Denis Burkitt published a study in which he noted that in countries where the population ate a diet high in fiber, cancer of colon and rectum—a leading cause of death in the United States— was relatively rare. Other studies have confirmed the link be- tween colorectal cancer and fiber. For example, a study at the Harvard School of Public Health recently examined the diets of seven thousand men. Researchers found that men who con- sumed the highest amount of saturated fat and the lowest amount of fiber were four times more likely to develop colon polyps, often a precursor to cancer.

Fiber may also offer protection against breast cancer, the second leading cause of cancer deaths among women. Studies have shown that women who develop breast cancer typically have higher levels of blood estrogen than women who remain cancer free. A recent study sponsored by the American Health Foundation attempted to see if fiber could lower blood estrogen levels. In the study, women were given 15 to 30 grams daily of wheat, corn, or oat bran. At the end of 2 months, the women on the wheat bran experienced a dramatic drop in blood estro- gen levels, but not the women on the other forms of fiber.

Heart Disease • Several studies have shown that soluble fiber can lower blood cholesterol levels, which decreases the risk of coronary artery disease and stroke. For example, psyl- lium, derived from the ground-up husks of the psyllium plant, is used as a laxative (Metamucil) and in cereal as a cholesterol- lowering agent. In fact, according to one study performed at the University of Kentucky Medical Service, a diet rich in psyllium flake cereal can reduce blood cholesterol levels by 12 percent. Based on this study, psyllium appears to be especially effective in lowering low-density lipoproteins, or "bad" cholesterol. (Psyllium can cause an allergic reaction in some people.)

Oat bran is another popular cholesterol buster. Studies show that by eating roughly three packets of instant oatmeal daily, you can cut your total cholesterol level by about six points, thus reducing your risk of heart attack.

Dried beans are also a potent cholesterol cutter. A recent study showed that by eating 4 ounces of cooked beans daily, people with cholesterol levels of over 200 milligrams per deciliter can reduce total cholesterol by as much as 20 percent.

Gastrointestinal Disorders • Insoluble fiber can help to ward off the kinds of gastrointestinal ailments that plague middle age and beyond. First, fiber can prevent constipation—infrequent bowel movements or hard stool that is difficult to pass. Constipation is not just uncomfortable, but it can promote *hemorrhoids*, varicose veins in the area of the anus and rectum. People with a chronic history of constipation are also more likely to develop diverticular disease (diverticulosis and diverticulitis), which affects more than one-third of all adults over fifty. *Diverticulosis* is characterized by the presence of diverticula, saclike herniations that can form in any part of the gastrointestinal tract, but more often than not in the colon. Symptoms of diverticulosis may vary from no symptoms at all to cramps, constipation, or diarrhea. Diverticulosis can develop into a more serious condition, *diverticulitis*, if the diverticula become inflamed. Diverticulosis is quite common among older people and is usually treated with a high-fiber diet. (Diverticulitis is treated with antibiotics and a low-fiber diet.)

Flax

FACTS

As far back as 8500 years ago, flax was a normal part of a diet that included other wild cereal grasses such as barley. In modern times, flax has been used primarily as a source of linen and linseed oil. Today, however, researchers at the National Cancer Institute are exploring the potential anticancer properties of an edible form of flaxseed. If their expectations are proven correct, flax may once again become a dietary mainstay.

THE RIGHT AMOUNT

Flaxseed oil is available as capsules or liquid at natural food stores. Take 1 to 3 capsules or 1 to 3 tablespoons daily. Ordinary flax can become rancid very quickly. Use only products that include stabilized flax. Vitamin-fortified, stabilized flaxseed baked products are available at some natural food stores and through mail order.

POSSIBLE BENEFITS

Cancer Fighter • Flax contains twenty-seven anticancer compounds including fiber, pectin, tocopherol (vitamin E), and sitosterol. Flax is also an excellent source of lignans, which are converted in the gut into compounds that are similar in structure to natural estrogens produced by the body. Lignans are believed to deactivate potent estrogens that can cause tumors to grow; like other phytoestrogens, they bind to estrogen receptor sites on cells in place of the more potent estrogens. Studies have shown that people who consume diets rich in lignans have lower levels of cancer of the breast and colon.

Folic Acid

FACTS

In recent years, pregnant women have been urged to take 400 micrograms of this B vitamin daily to prevent neural tube defects in their babies. But folic acid is not just for the very young—it's for people of all ages, especially those who want to live to be a ripe old age.

Folic acid helps in the formation of red blood cells and in nucleic acids, RNA and DNA, the genetic material in the cells.

Folic acid is derived from the word *foliage* because it is found in dark green leafy vegetables such as spinach and broccoli. It is also found in dried beans, frozen orange juice, yeast, liver, sunflower seeds, wheat germ, and fortified breakfast cereals.

THE RIGHT AMOUNT

The recommended daily allowance for folic acid is 400 micrograms, roughly the amount in 1½ cups of boiled spinach or ½ cup of peanuts. Women on average get only one-half of the recommended daily allowance. Supplements of 400 micrograms are sometimes supplied in B-complex formulas. One hundred micrograms of folic acid is the usual amount found in supplements.

POSSIBLE BENEFITS

Heart Disease • Folic acid may help to prevent the number one killer of both men and women in the United States—heart disease—by helping to maintain normal levels of homocysteine, an amino acid found in the body. In a recent study performed at Harvard Medical School, men with even a *slightly* elevated level of homocysteine were three times more likely to have a heart attack than men with the lowest levels. Based on the study, when given a folic acid supplement, homocysteine levels dropped back to normal in most men. Researchers at Harvard say that patients who are believed to be at high risk of having a heart attack should have their homocysteine levels checked. Here's my advice: even if you're not at high risk of having a heart attack, it just makes good sense to eat a diet rich in folic acid.

Cancer Fighter • Researchers at Brigham and Women's Hospital in Boston have linked a diet low in folic acid to a change in DNA that may allow cancer-causing genes to be expressed. In their study of 26,000 men and women, those with the lowest intake of folic acid had the highest level of adenomas (precancerous tumors) of the colon or rectum. At Tufts University, researchers are studying whether very high does of folate—about twenty times the current recommended level of 400 micrograms—can help prevent colon cancer in people with precancerous polyps.

Low levels of folic acid have also been linked to cervical cancer. Each year, 6000 women die of cervical cancer in the United States. Cervical dysplasia—cell abnormalities that if left untreated, often lead to cancer—can be caused by an infection with the human papillomavirus. (Cigarette smoking, multiple sex partners, and early age at first intercourse are also believed to increase the risk of cervical cancer.) In a recent study performed at the University of Alabama, 300 women with cervical dysplasia were compared with 170 healthy women. These women were interviewed about their lifestyle and eating habits. As part of the study, blood levels for certain vitamins were also checked. The results: women with the highest levels of folic acid had the lowest levels of cervical dysplasia, even if they were infected with the human papillomavirus. The researchers concluded that folic acid may offer some protection against this potentially lethal virus.

Fo-ti

FACTS

According to Chinese legend, this herb (known as *ho shou wu* in China) can help prevent hair from turning gray. Fo-ti is a favorite longevity herb among Chinese herbalists. Although there is little evidence to prove that fo-ti can help maintain hair color, recent studies show that this herb may offer real protection against heart disease.

THE RIGHT AMOUNT

Fo-ti is available as capsules at natural food stores. Take 1 capsule up to three times daily.

POSSIBLE BENEFITS

Heart Disease • Several Chinese studies have shown that fo-ti can lower blood cholesterol levels, thus helping to protect against heart attack. In addition, this herb contains flavonoid-like compounds that strengthen and dilate blood vessels, improving the flow of blood to the heart.

PERSONAL ADVICE

The Chinese have a mystical reverence for fo-ti. According to Chinese folklore, the older the root, the more powerful its rejuvenating properties!

Gamma-linolenic Acid

FACTS

Gamma-linolenic acid (GLA) is a fatty acid that is extracted from the seeds of evening primrose or borage plants. For centuries, herbalists have valued both plants for their medicinal properties. Today, GLA is marketed as evening primrose oil and can be found in most natural food stores. GLA is a very popular over-the-counter treatment in Canada and Europe (especially Britain) for a wide range of ailments ranging from premenstrual syndrome to skin rashes. Recent studies suggest that GLA may help prevent cardiovascular disease, provide relief for rheumatoid arthritis, and may even be used one day as a cancer treatment.

THE RIGHT AMOUNT

GLA is available in capsule form. Take 250 milligrams up to three times daily.

POSSIBLE BENEFITS

Reduces Inflammation   •   In a study reported in the November 1, 1993, issue of *Annals of Internal Medicine*, researchers at the University of Pennsylvania's Graduate Hospital in Philadelphia gave capsules containing 1.4 grams of GLA daily to nineteen people with rheumatoid arthritis (RA), an autoimmune disorder characterized by inflamed and painful joints. Eighteen other RA patients received a placebo. After six months, the group on the

GLA showed less pain and less signs of inflammation than the patients taking the placebo. The research team did not find any adverse side effects associated with GLA. More studies need to be done to see if GLA is an effective treatment for RA.

Heart Disease   •   Several studies have shown that GLA may lower cholesterol levels in some people. In one Canadian study, patients taking 4 grams of evening primrose oil daily experienced a 31.5 percent decline in cholesterol after 3 months. However, other studies have shown that GLA has only a small effect on lowering cholesterol.

In a study conducted at McMaster University in Hamilton, Canada, researchers tested GLA's ability to prevent blood clots. Rabbits were fed various fatty acids, including GLA, for a 4-week period. The researchers found that GLA appears to inhibit platelets (blood cells involved in the formation of blood clots) from adhering to the walls of blood vessels. Thus, GLA may help to prevent blood clots, a major cause of heart attack and stroke.

Cancer Fighter   •   A recent study performed at Nazam's Institute of Medical Sciences in India has shown that GLA can selectively kill tumor cells. In a clinical trial, six patients with gliomas, a particular type of tumor, were given GLA. All the patients showed mild improvement. This doesn't mean that GLA is a cure for cancer; however, one day GLA may prove to be an effective treatment in conjunction with other therapies against certain types of tumors.

Genistein

FACTS

Genistein is a hot "new" anticancer compound that's actually been around for thousands of years, but until recently, nobody has noticed. Genistein is a recently identified isoflavone found in soy and soy-based products. For decades, scientists have been mystified as to why the incidence of many different forms of cancer in Asia is so much lower than in the United States. (For example, the breast cancer rate in the United States is 22.4 per 100,000; in Japan it's 6 per 100,000.) Recent studies suggest that genistein could be a potent cancer fighter.

Good sources of genistein include whole soy beans, tofu (bean curd), soy flour, soy milk, and rehydrated vegetable protein, which can be used in place of chopped meat in foods such as tacos and chili. (Soy sauce does not contain genistein.)

THE RIGHT AMOUNT

Eat one or two portions of soy foods per day (about 3 ounces).

POSSIBLE BENEFITS

Cancer Fighter • Since 1987, several hundred papers have been published on genistein's role as a possible cancer fighter. In 1993, a German study published in *The Proceedings of the National Academy of Sciences* found that in test tube studies, genistein blocks a process called *angiogenesis*, which is responsible for the growth of new blood vessels. The researchers speculate that genistein may indirectly prevent the growth of tumors by thwarting the formation of new blood vessels that are necessary to nourish them. In other words, genistein literally starves little tumors before they can grow into bigger problems. The researchers go on to note that in animal studies, soy products have inhibited the formation of mammary tumors, and they logically conclude that genistein may be the compound protecting Japanese women from breast cancer.

Autopsies of Japanese men show that prostate cancer is as common among Japanese men as it is among American men, but the cancer seems to grow much more slowly, so slowly in fact, that many die without ever developing clinical disease. Until recently, there was no explanation for this phenomenon. However, researchers now suspect that genistein is actually blocking the growth of these tumors. Finnish researcher Herman Aldercreutz and colleagues compared blood plasma levels of isoflavones in Japanese and Finnish men. The levels of isoflavones were more than 100 times higher among the Japanese men, with genistein occurring in the highest concentration of any other isoflavone. The researchers concluded "a life-long high concentration of isoflavonoids in plasma (Japanese children have as high a urinary excretion as adults) might explain why Japanese men have small latent carcinomas that seldom develop to clinical disease" (*The Lancet*, November 13, 1993).

Researchers Greg Peterson and Stephen Barnes of the University of Alabama tested whether genistein could block the growth of non-estrogen-dependent human breast cancer cells. In this study, they showed that genistein thwarted the growth of breast cancer in vitro and that the presence of an estrogen receptor is not necessary for isoflavones to inhibit tumor growth. This suggests that the protective effect of isoflavones may not be due to their effect on hormones, but rather, the particular ability of genistein to block cell growth.

Genistein holds great promise as a potential cancer protector. However, more studies need to be done to confirm whether this is true.

Heart Disease • Genistein is believed to inhibit the action of enzymes that may promote cell growth and migration. Some researchers speculate that by blocking the action of these enzymes, genistein may also prevent the growth of cells that form plaque deposits in arteries, much the same way that genistein may prevent the growth of tumors.

Ginger

FACTS

Ginger root is one of the most widely used herbs in the world. In China, where it is highly regarded as a "warming herb," it was mentioned in the famous *Shen Nung Herbal*, which dates back to 3000 B.C. Ginger is also a major medicinal herb in Ayurvedic medicine, the Indian system of traditional medicine, which is rapidly gaining popularity in the West. In the United States, the National Cancer Institute has included ginger in its Experimental Food Program, which is exploring the cancer preventive compounds in different foods.

Herbal healers in the West have long prescribed ginger as a treatment for nausea and morning sickness.

THE RIGHT AMOUNT

Fresh ginger is sold at supermarkets and greengrocers. It can be used in cooking or made into a tea. Ginger capsules and teas are available at natural food stores. Take 1 capsule up to three times daily, or drink 1 to 2 cups of ginger tea.

POSSIBLE BENEFITS

Cancer Fighter   •   Ginger is abundant in a compound called *geraniol*, which may be a potent cancer fighter. In a recent study, Dr. Charles Ellson of the University of Wisconsin, Nutrition Science Department, found that only 0.1 percent of geraniol increased the survival rate of rats with malignant tumors. In addition, studies have shown that geraniol can enhance the effectiveness of other anticancer drugs. More studies are being done to determine if geraniol will have similar effects on people.

Heart Disease   •   Several studies have shown that ginger can prevent platelet aggregation, that is, it can prevent blood cells from sticking together and forming blood clots. If a clot lodges in an artery leading to the heart or the brain, it can cause a heart attack or stroke. In one Indian study, twenty healthy male volunteers were fed 100 grams of butter daily, which significantly increased their rate of platelet aggregation. However, when ten of the men were given 5 grams of dry ginger divided into two doses with the fatty meal, the ginger appeared to inhibit the degree of platelet aggregation.

Migraine   •   A Danish study showed that ginger may help prevent migraine headaches, and may relieve some of the symptoms of these headaches such as pain and nausea. Studies show that ginger has anti-inflammatory activity, which could explain why it would work as a pain reliever.

Ginkgo

FACTS

Do you have difficulty remembering the names of people even if you've just been introduced to them? Do you find yourself becoming more forgetful? Becoming forgetful is one of the most negative stereotypes of aging, and the bad news is, there's some truth to it. A recent survey of nearly fifteen thousand adults over age fifty-five revealed that about three-quarters of them had some difficulty remembering things. The good news is, the leaf from an ancient tree may help to perk up your memory. Recent studies suggest that extract from the ginkgo tree leaf may help improve memory, maintain mental sharpness, and provide many other life-extending benefits.

The ginkgo tree, which dates back to before the Ice Age, is one of the hardiest trees known to humankind. Some live as long as four thousand years! Although the ginkgo kernel has been used in Oriental medicine for hundreds of years, it was only in the 1970s that European researchers began investigating the potential medicinal properties of the ginkgo leaf. Today, ginkgo is one of the most commonly prescribed drugs in Europe for a wide range of problems ranging from memory loss to tinnitus (ringing in the ears) to hemorrhoids to headaches.

Although ginkgo products are sold in natural food stores, ginkgo may soon be used as a serious drug in the United States. In 1988, a chemist at Harvard synthesized a ginkgo compound called *ginkgolide B*, which, among other things, is being tested as a potential drug for asthma and to help prevent the rejection of transplanted organs.

THE RIGHT AMOUNT

Ginkgo, which is growing in popularity, is available in most natural food stores and even many drug stores. I recommend a supplement called Ginkgo 24 containing a solution of 24 percent ginkgo biloba in a 50:1 extract. Take 60-milligram capsules or tablets three times daily. The effects of ginkgo are short-lived—the dose lasts for only a few hours. There is no known toxicity.

POSSIBLE BENEFITS

Memory Booster • There are several reasons why older adults may have difficulty remembering. Stress, lack of physical exercise, poor mental stimulation, and even subtle vitamin deficiencies may impair cognitive function. However, there is also a natural slowing down in mental processes due to decreased levels of certain chemicals in the brain. Electrical impulses or messages from the brain are transmitted along nerve cells called *neurons*. Neurons have long tendrils called *axons*, which overlap onto another neuron. Neurons "communicate" with each other via chemicals called *neurotransmitters*, notably dopamine and noradrenaline. As we age, there is a decreased production of neurotransmitters, thus resulting in reduced alertness and memory retention. Animal studies have shown that ginkgo increases the level of dopamine, which improves the body's ability to transmit information. Several human studies have shown that ginkgo can improve mental performance among elderly people who have shown deteriorating mental function. Studies of younger people suggest that high doses of ginkgo can improve short-term mental processes. In his book, *Next Generation Herbal Medicine,* herbalist Daniel Mowrey, Ph.D., suggested that one day, college students may use ginkgo to help them cram for exams.

Improves Circulation • Studies also show that ginkgo improves the blood flow to the brain (and to other vital organs), providing oxygen and nutrients the brain needs to function at peak capacity. As we age, circulation is often impaired by plaque deposits in the arteries delivering blood to the brain and other organs. Ginkgo helps to dilate or relax arteries and veins, thus improving blood flow throughout the body.

Antioxidant • Ginkgo is rich in flavonoids, potent antioxidants that protect the body against free radicals or unstable molecules that can cause damage to healthy cells. Heart disease, cancer, and even arthritis are just some of the diseases that are believed to be caused or worsened by free radical damage.

Prevents Blood Clots • Studies show that ginkgo inhibits blood cells from sticking together, thus preventing the formation of blood clots that can lead to heart attack or stroke. (If a clot lodges in an artery leading to the heart, it can cause a heart attack. If it lodges in an artery leading to the brain, it can cause a stroke.)

PERSONAL ADVICE

Try taking ginkgo capsules for hemorrhoids. Many people swear that is it is one of the most effective agents for helping to control bleeding and itching due to irritated hemorrhoids.

Ginseng

FACTS

Of all the substances listed in the anti-aging hot hundred, ginseng may be the most widely used. For five thousand years, the Chinese have revered this herb as a cure-all for nearly every ailment, from impotence to heart disease, and as an overall antidote to the ravages of aging. In recent years, ginseng has been promoted in the West as a tonic and a rejuvenator, which has generated a great deal of interest in this herb. At last count, there were more than three thousand scientific studies performed on ginseng. Most of these studies were done in the Orient or in the former Soviet Union, where ginseng (a home-grown variety) is routinely given to athletes to improve stamina and performance. Although more research needs to be done, there is strong evidence that ginseng has many positive effects on the body and the mind.

There are three different types of ginseng: panax ginseng is grown in China; American ginseng (*Panax quinquefolius*) is grown in the United States. Siberian ginseng (*Eleutherococcus senticosus*), grown in Siberia, is actually not ginseng at all, but a close relative that has similar affects. All forms of ginseng have similar properties, with some differences. Chinese ginseng is considered the strongest form of ginseng; American ginseng is milder and is highly prized in the Orient.

THE RIGHT AMOUNT

Ginseng comes in many forms including capsules, tea, and powder. I recommend American or Siberian ginseng; some people may find panax ginseng too stimulating, especially at night. For capsules, take 1 up to three times daily. For tea, drink 1 cup daily. If you use powder, mix 5 to 10 grams in liquid daily. Excess use of ginseng can make some people very jittery; do not exceed the recommended dose.

Caution: In rare cases, ginseng, which has a mildly estrogenic effect on the body, can cause vaginal bleeding in postmenopausal women. If this happens, be sure to tell your doctor that you are using ginseng; vaginal bleeding can be mistaken as a symptom of uterine cancer. Do not use ginseng if you have high blood pressure or an irregular heartbeat.

Be sure to buy ginseng products from a reputable company. Ginseng is expensive, and many unscrupulous distributors may try to pass off cheaper products as ginseng.

POSSIBLE BENEFITS

Stimulant • Oriental healers contend that ginseng improves mental performance, especially in older people. Animal studies confirm that ginseng may improve the capacity to learn. For example, rats given ginseng were able to run through a maze faster to find a food reward than were untreated rats. Several human studies found that people taking ginseng made fewer mistakes and may even complete tasks faster than people not taking ginseng. There are several theories as to why ginseng may have a positive effect on learning. Some researchers speculate that ginseng may indirectly stimulate the production of stress hormones that can increase stamina and prevent fatigue. However, ginseng also contains choline, a chemical in the brain that is essential for learning and memory retention, which may also help to perk up mental activity (see Choline, p.52). More studies are needed to determine ginseng's exact effect on mental functioning.

Antioxidant • Ginseng contains antioxidants, substances that prevent cellular damage due to oxidation, exposure to unstable molecules called free radicals. Free radicals are believed to be responsible for promoting mutations in cells that could lead to cancer. In addition, free radicals may play a role in heart disease by promoting the formation of low-density lipoproteins, or "bad" cholesterol.

Cancer Fighter • Researchers at Japan's Kanazawa University found that unpurified saponins, compounds found in ginseng, inhibited the growth of cancer cells and actually converted diseased cells into normal cells.

Lowers Cholesterol • Japanese researchers showed that rats who were fed a high-cholesterol diet showed a drop in cholesterol and a rise in beneficial high-density lipoprotein, or "good" cholesterol, after being fed ginseng.

Antistress • Soviet scientist I. I. Brekhman, Ph.D., first coined the term *adaptogen* to describe ginseng. According to studies performed by Brekhman, ginseng helps the body to better cope with stress by normalizing body functions. For example, if blood sugar levels drop too low or blood pressure rises too high, Brekhman contends that ginseng somehow brings the body back to normal levels. Although the concept of an adaptogen may seem foreign to Westerners who take medication only when they are sick, it is in keeping with traditional Chinese medicine, which uses ginseng and other herbs as a tonic to maintain overall health.

Menopause • Ginseng contains compounds that are similar in action to estrogen, the female sex hormone. Many women use ginseng to help control some of the unpleasant side effects of menopause, such as hot flashes, which may occur when estrogen levels decline. (Interestingly enough, in countries where ginseng is commonly used, such as China and Japan, menopause is not considered a "medical problem," nor do post-menopausal women routinely take estrogen supplements.)

PERSONAL ADVICE

Take ginseng 1 hour before eating. Vitamin C can interfere with the absorption of ginseng, so if you take a C supplement, wait 2 hours before or after taking ginseng to do so.

Glutathione

FACTS

I call glutathione the "triple-threat anti-aging amino acid" because it is synthesized from three amino acids: L-cysteine, L-glutamic acid, and glycine, all of which are found in fruits and vegetables. Glutathione is a potent antioxidant that is synthesized by our own body cells. Studies have shown that glutathione may help protect against cancer, radiation poisoning, and the detrimental effects of cigarette smoke and alcohol abuse. Glutathione is a popular supplement in Japan, the country with the longest life span in the world. Although many mainstream U.S. scientists have dismissed glutathione supplements as worthless, a recent study sponsored by the Human Nutrition Research Center on Aging at Tufts University suggests that glutathione supplements may help keep an aging immune system healthy.

THE RIGHT AMOUNT

Glutathione is present in fruits and vegetables; however, cooking can reduce its potency. I recommend taking 50-milligram capsules one or two times daily.

POSSIBLE BENEFITS

Immune Booster   •   Simin N. Meydani, Ph.D., a well-known researcher in the field of nutrition who discovered that vitamin E had a positive effect on the immune system of elderly people, investigated whether glutathione would have a similar effect on aging white blood cells in animals and humans. In both animal and human studies, Dr. Meydani found glutathione gave the immune system a much-needed boost. It not only improved the blood cells' ability to produce substances that can help ward off infection, but it also reduced the amount of inflammatory substances produced by the cells. Interestingly enough, glutathione had a greater effect on the sluggish cells of older people than on younger ones. More research needs to be done before we can say that glutathione is a bona fide immune booster, but the preliminary evidence looks good.

Anti-inflammatory   •   Glutathione has been used as treatment for allergies and arthritis, both conditions that are caused by an inflammatory response in the body.

PERSONAL ADVICE

Here's more evidence that when it comes to aging well, the adage Use it or lose it! takes on new importance. Studies suggest that exercise may increase the level of antioxidants such as glutathione in older people.

Grapeseed Extract

FACTS

Grapeseed extract is touted as a potent anti-aging compound in France, and is fast gaining popularity in the United States.

Grapeseed extract contains a unique type of bioflavonoids called *proanthocyanidins*, which are synergistic with vitamin C, that is, they greatly enhance the activity of vitamin C. In fact, some researchers believe that grapeseed extract helps vitamin C enter cells, thus strengthening the cell membranes and protecting the cells from oxidative damage.

Proanthocyanidins are also found in cranberries, cola nuts, and other fruits and vegetables.

THE RIGHT AMOUNT

Grapeseed extract is sold in capsule form at natural food stores. Take 1–2 (30–100 milligrams) of grapeseed extract daily.

POSSIBLE BENEFITS

Cancer Fighter • Grapeseed extract is a potent antioxidant and free radical scavenger. Free radicals are unstable oxygen molecules that can attack normal cells, destroying them or causing them to mutate. Free radical damage can also lead to the kind of unfettered cell growth associated with cancer. Vitamin C is a potent antioxidant in its own right, but studies suggest that it may be even more effective when combined with proanthocyanidins such as grapeseed extract. In fact, according to researchers at the Department of Pharmacy of Nagasaki University School of Medicine in Japan, test tube studies showed that the bioflavonoids in grapeseed extract had stronger antioxidant activity than vitamin C.

Heart Disease • Several studies have confirmed that antioxidants like grapeseed extract can prevent the oxidation of blood lipids, such as low-density lipoprotein, or "bad" cholesterol, which can promote the formation of plaque or fatty deposits in the arteries.

Anti-inflammatory • Grapeseed extract has been used as an anti-inflammatory to treat common ailments such as arthritis and allergies. Many bioflavonoids inhibit the release of certain enzymes that can promote inflammation. In the case of arthritis, free radical damage may also contribute to joint pain and swelling associated with this condition.

Circulation • Capillaries are tiny blood vessels that can be easily destroyed by free radical damage. In addition, as we age, cells lose collagen, a protein fiber that is important for the growth and repair of cells including capillary cells. Weakened capillaries can lead to easy bruising and a tendency to develop varicose veins. Grapeseed extract helps strengthen capillaries in two ways. By protecting against free radical assault, grapeseed extract may help prevent weakening of capillaries. In addition, since vitamin C is essential for the production of collagen and grapeseed extract enhances the performance of vitamin C, it is indirectly involved in collagen production.

Green Tea

FACTS

If there was an Olympic competition for longevity, the Japanese would be the world champions. The Japanese have a longer life span than any other nationality, even though they are heavy smokers. What's their secret? Some researchers in the United States and Japan are looking for the answer in a cup of tea—no, they're not reading tea leaves, they're reading some impressive studies that suggest that phytochemicals found in green tea may help fight against cancer and heart disease.

Green tea, derived from the tea plant, is a rich source of potentially beneficial compounds called *catechins*. As tea undergoes processing, it loses some of its precious catechins to oxidation. Green tea is very lightly processed, thus retaining more of its catechins than the heavily processed dry black tea that is sold in the United States.

THE RIGHT AMOUNT

Sip 1 or 2 cups of green tea daily. Real green tea is found in natural food stores or Asian markets. Green tea extract tablets are also available. Take 1–2 tablets daily.

POSSIBLE BENEFITS

Cancer Fighter • Researchers at the American Health Foundation in New York exposed mice to nitrosamines, a potent cancer-causing agent in cigarette smoke. One group of exposed mice was given green tea, the other was not. The results: there were 45 percent fewer cases of lung cancer among the teetotaling mice. In other studies of lab mice, green tea helped to slow the rate of tumor growth in mice exposed to ultraviolet radiation.

Does this mean that green tea will work as well in humans? There's some evidence that it might. The cancer rate in central Japan is lower than anywhere else in Japan; coincidentally, it is the place where green tea is produced and where the people drink more of the stuff than anywhere else in the country. More studies remain to be done before we'll know for sure whether or not green tea is a bona fide cancer protector; however, drinking a cup or two of tea a day can't hurt and just may help.

Cholesterol Buster • Animal studies show that green tea catechins can reduce cholesterol levels in laboratory rats fed a diet high in saturated fat and cholesterol. Human studies have shown that people who eat a high-cholesterol diet (averaging three egg yolks in one meal) can maintain normal cholesterol levels by sipping green tea with their meals. I'm not suggesting that green tea will work this well for everyone or that you can eat a high-fat diet as long as you wash it down with green tea. However, adding green tea to an already sensible diet may be a good way to keep cholesterol levels in check.

PERSONAL ADVICE

Coffee drinkers take note: on average, brewed tea contains one-half the caffeine found in coffee and is probably twice as good for you.

Hawthorn

FACTS

Heart disease is the number one killer of both men and women in the United States, which is why I believe this "heart healthy" herb will become very hot as the baby boom generation reaches middle age and beyond.

Since the 1700s, European herbalists have used preparations made from the hawthorn plant as a tonic for the heart. Today, this herb is widely used throughout Europe, notably in France, England, Russia, and Germany, and is gaining in popularity in the United States.

THE RIGHT AMOUNT

Hawthorn is available in capsule form or as a tea at natural food stores. Take 1 capsule up to three times daily. (Preparations sold in the United States are made from the hawthorn berry.) Drink 1 to 3 cups of tea daily.

Caution: If you are on any medication for your heart, do not discontinue or alter your dose without talking with your physician or healer.

POSSIBLE BENEFITS

Heart Disease   •   Hawthorn is a well-researched herb, especially in Europe. Animal and human studies show that hawthorn has many positive effects on the cardiovascular system. Hawthorn is rich in bioflavonoids, compounds that strengthen capillaries, thus improving the flow of blood throughout the body. Studies on humans and dogs have shown that hawthorn can reduce blood pressure during exertion; animal studies also show that this herb can increase the contractility of the heart muscle, strengthening the heart's ability to pump blood. In fact, in Europe, hawthorn may be prescribed along with the drug digitalis to regulate the heartbeat; the addition of hawthorn reduces the required dose of digitalis. Other studies have shown that hawthorn may be useful as a treatment for angina (chest pain due to insufficient blood flow to the heart) and may also decrease the heartbeat rate, preventing the heart from becoming overworked. Many natural healers believe that hawthorn can keep an aging heart pumping like a young one!

Horsetail

FACTS

Horsetail is a bamboolike plant that lives in marshes which has been used for hundreds of years by herbal healers as a treatment for rheumatoid arthritis. This herb is also a mild diuretic; it is used by homeopathic physicians as a remedy for urinary problems and enlarged prostate. There is a growing interest in herbs such as horsetail these days due to the aging population and the rise in age-related ailments such as arthritis and prostate problems.

THE RIGHT AMOUNT

Horsetail is available as tablets or capsules at natural food stores. Take up to 3 tablets or capsules daily. Some studies show that very high doses of horsetail have been toxic to livestock. However, the low doses recommended here should not have any adverse affects.

POSSIBLE BENEFITS

Rheumatoid Arthritis • Gold shots are a traditional remedy for rheumatoid arthritis. Horsetail has been shown to absorb minute quantities of gold that are dissolved in water. Some herbalists believe that the gold residue in horsetail may be the reason why some people find it effective against the joint pain and stiffness associated with arthritis.

Hair Enhancer • The Meskawki Indians fed horsetail to their ponies to improve the gloss of their hair. Horsetail is rich in silica, a mineral that is reputed to add shine and strength to hair. In fact, it is used in many shampoos and conditioners. Silica is also used to strengthen nails.

Legumes

FACTS

Legumes (dried beans and peas) are a mainstay of many diets around the world, although not in the United States. Rice and beans is a staple south of the border; *pasta e fagioli* (pasta and beans) is standard fare in Italy. Maybe not so coincidentally, people who live in countries where legumes are a major part of their cuisine have substantially lower rates of cancer and heart disease.

Legumes include all kinds of beans, ranging from kidney to navy to lentil to black beans. All legumes are pretty much the same nutritionally, although there are some slight variations in fiber content and caloric value. Legumes are an excellent source of protein; however, most lack certain essential amino acids that are found in meat (soybeans are the exception—they contain all eight essential amino acids that cannot be produced by the body). The amino acids that are missing in legumes are present in grains; therefore, by eating legumes with a grain such as rice, you can create a meal containing all eight essential amino acids.

THE RIGHT AMOUNT

I recommend eating at least three legume-based meals weekly.

POSSIBLE BENEFITS

Cancer Fighter • Legumes contain many compounds that are believed to protect against cancer. Legumes are a good source of *isoflavones,* compounds that block estrogen receptors in some cells and by doing so may deactivate potent forms of estrogen that can trigger the growth of estrogen-dependent tumor cells. About 30 percent of all breast tumors are estrogen dependent.

Legumes are also rich in *protease inhibitors,* compounds that block the action of enzymes that can trigger cancer growth, and *phytic acid,* compounds that in animal studies have been shown to thwart the growth of tumors.

Legumes are an excellent source of *fiber,* substances in plants that are not digested and absorbed by the body. A diet high in fiber is believed to protect against some forms of cancer, particularly cancer of the colon. No one knows exactly how fiber helps to prevent cancer, however, one theory is that fiber moves food more quickly through the colon. As food is broken down into its basic components, potential carcinogens are released into the gut. Some carcinogens may be naturally occurring; some may be from insecticides or added in processing. If food is speeded through the gastrointestinal tract, there is less exposure to these potential cancer threats.

Lowers Cholesterol • A study at the University of Kentucky showed that legumes are powerful cholesterol busters. Eating 4 ounces of cooked beans daily (1 cup) can over time reduce cholesterol levels of over 200 milligrams per deciliter by as much as 20 percent!

Diabetes • As we age, we are much more likely to develop insulin resistance, that is, the body becomes less efficient at metabolizing or utilizing glucose (blood sugar). High levels of blood sugar are associated with diabetes, which increases the risk of heart attack, stroke, and other vascular problems. Many researchers believe that diet may help to prevent diabetes, or at least delay its onset in some people. Notably, foods that avoid a heavy concentration of sugar in the bloodstream at one time may be better than foods that force insulin to work overtime. Complex carbohydrates, the kind found in legumes and grains, are just what the doctor ordered. They burn slowly and steadily in the body (not like sweets, which burn very quickly), thus giving the insulin the time it needs to utilize glucose.

Lemongrass

FACTS

Lemongrass is one of many foods that is widely used in Asian cuisines but virtually nonexistent in American cooking. Also known as *citronella*, lemongrass adds a fresh, lemony flavor to food. It's not only delicious, but studies show that lemongrass oil may help protect against heart disease by lowering cholesterol.

Fresh lemongrass and lemongrass oil is sold in Asian markets and natural food stores. If using the whole plant, the lower part of the stalk is crushed and finely chopped. Lemongrass oil is used as a flavoring.

THE RIGHT AMOUNT

Use the plant or the oil in cooking whenever you can. Add one stalk of chopped lemongrass to stir-fry vegetables and other Oriental dishes. Many Oriental recipes call for lemongrass oil.

POSSIBLE BENEFITS

Heart Disease • Researchers at the University of Wisconsin gave men with high cholesterol 140 milligrams of lemongrass oil daily for 3 months. At the end of the study, 30 percent of the men experienced a 10 percent decrease in cholesterol. The researchers suspect that a compound in lemongrass decreases the synthesis of cholesterol from fats.

Licorice

FACTS

When Westerners think of licorice, they think of the licorice-flavored candy that contains little if any of the real herb. In China, however, licorice is the mostly widely used of all medicinal herbs. Five thousand years ago, licorice was immortalized in the famous *Shen Nung Herbal.* Today in China, licorice is highly regarded as a tonic and longevity herb. Recently, licorice's potential health benefits have attracted the attention of Western scientists; it is currently under investigation by the National Cancer Institute for its possible anticancer properties.

THE RIGHT AMOUNT

Take 1 capsule up to three times daily.

Caution: Licorice should not be used by people with high blood pressure.

POSSIBLE BENEFITS

Menopause • Licorice is frequently used to treat symptoms of menopause. Licorice contains a glycyrrhizin, a hormonelike compound that appears to help normalize hormone levels in women.

Cancer Fighter • Animal studies show that glycyrrhetinic acid (derived from glycyrrhizin) can block carcinogen-induced tumor growth. More studies are being done to determine if licorice is an anticancer herb.

Arthritis • Due to its anti-inflammatory action, herbal healers prescribe licorice to treat the swelling, aches, and pains of arthritis.

Antiulcer • Carbendoxolane, a compound found in licorice, has been used successfully to treat stomach ulcers.

Lignans

FACTS

People who live in countries where plant food is a mainstay of the diet, such as in Asia and Africa, have a much lower rate of many forms of cancer than people who live in Western countries where the diet is heavy in meat and light on fruits and vegetables.

For several decades, researchers have attempted to isolate the specific components in plant food that may help to prevent various diseases. Scientists have studied various vitamins, minerals, and fiber, the nondigestible food substance in plants that is not digested by the body. Each of these substances may play a role; however, some may play a greater role than others. In 1979, scientists discovered a compound in fiber called *lignans*, and today, many researchers believe that lignans may be responsible for much of fiber's protective effect.

Many studies have shown that lignans have anticarcinogenic, antiviral, and antifungal properties. They are also rich in phytoestrogens, hormonelike compounds that mimic the behavior of natural hormones in the body.

Flaxseed is the best plant source of lignans. However, wheat bran and rye also have these compounds. Smaller amounts of lignans can be found in many plants and vegetables.

THE RIGHT AMOUNT

Research on lignans is relatively new; therefore, we have no idea of the precise amount that is needed to prevent cancer. I recommend eating foods that are rich in lignans, such as grains, fruits, and vegetables. Bread made from flax is a particularly good source of lignans and can be found at many natural food stores.

POSSIBLE BENEFITS

Cancer Fighter • There are several theories on why lignans may protect against cancer. Studies have shown that vegetarian and semivegetarian women have a much lower rate of breast cancer than women who eat meat. Researchers have measured the amount of lignans and estrogen in the urine of vegetarian women and have found that their urine contained higher amounts of both estrogen and lignans than women who were not vegetarians. What was even more interesting was the fact that women who had breast cancer excreted much smaller amounts of lignans and estrogen in their urine than either vegetarians or meat eaters and had higher blood levels of estrogen. From these studies, researchers suspected that lignans had a protective effect against breast cancer.

Other studies have shown that lignans are converted into estrogenlike compounds in the body that mimic the behavior of estrogen. Some forms of naturally produced estrogen are believed to promote the growth of estrogen-sensitive tumors. Certain cells in the body have receptors that bind with estrogen. Lignans, which are chemically similar to estrogen, may compete with the more potent natural forms of estrogen for space on estrogen-sensitive cells. If natural estrogen has no place to bind, it becomes deactivated, thus losing its ability to promote the growth of tumors. Excess estrogen is excreted in urine.

Some researchers believe that lignans may also be protective against cancer of the prostate and colon.

Ligusticum

FACTS

Ligusticum (licidum or wallichii) is an important Chinese herb that is in hot demand in the West because of its reputation as an immune booster. This herb, combined with astralagus, reishi, and other immune herbs, is used by natural healers to strengthen compromised immune systems (as in the case of AIDS patients or cancer patients receiving chemotherapy).

Ligusticum is a highly revered herb in China and is used in a famous woman's tonic called Four Things Soup, which includes dong quai. (See p. 68.)

There are more than sixty species of ligusticum worldwide. In the southwestern United States, Native Americans have long used *Ligusticum porteri* to treat viral, fungal, and respiratory infections. In the United States, ligusticum is marketed as osha and can be found in most natural food stores.

THE RIGHT AMOUNT

Osha and ligusticum are sold as capsules and extract at natural food stores. Take 2 or 3 capsules daily, or 5 to 10 drops of extract in liquid two or three times daily.

POSSIBLE BENEFITS

Cancer Fighter • Many species of ligusticum have been shown to inhibit the growth of tumors in animals.

Cardiovascular • A stroke can occur if the flow of blood to the brain is impaired in any way. There have been many studies investigating ligusticum and its role in the prevention of stroke. Several animal studies performed in China show that ligusticum can promote circulation to the brain and prevent the formation of blood clots. When a stroke was induced in animal tests, ligusticum helped restore circulation to the brain, thus minimizing brain damage. In fact, one Chinese study involving 158 patients with transient ischemic attack (tiny strokes) showed that ligusticum was even more effective than aspirin in helping to resolve blood clots and improve blood flow to the brain.

In China, ligusticum has also been used to treat angina, a condition that is caused by a reduction in blood flow to the heart.

Lutein

FACTS

Lutein is a member of the carotenoid family, a group of six hundred compounds naturally occurring in fruits and vegetables (of which beta-carotene is the most well known). Carotenoids are believed to offer special protection against many different forms of cancer, and recent studies suggest that lutein may also be a cancer fighter. Carotenoids provide fruits and vegetables with their orange, red, and yellow colors. However, they are also found in green leafy vegetables, but they are hidden by the green color of chlorophyll.

Good sources of lutein are spinach; greens, such as collard, turnip, and mustard; broccoli; green peas; celery; and kale.

THE RIGHT AMOUNT

There is no recommended daily allowance for lutein; however, I recommend eating one serving of a lutein-rich vegetable daily.

POSSIBLE BENEFITS

Cancer Fighter • A recent study of twelve hundred people performed at the University of Hawaii found that people who ate foods high in lutein had a lower risk of lung cancer than those who ate lower levels of lutein. Researchers suspect that lutein's anticancer properties are due to its antioxidant action.

Population studies have linked a high intake of fruits and vegetables that are rich in carotenoids with a lower risk of cancers of the head, neck, lung, esophagus, and colon.

Lycopene

FACTS

Lycopene, a member of the carotenoid family, is a potent antioxidant that may prove to be one of the most important of all the phytochemicals.

Lycopene, which gives fruits and vegetables a reddish color, is found primarily in tomato, ruby red grapefruit, and red peppers.

THE RIGHT AMOUNT

Eat one lycopene-rich food daily. Lycopene (along with other phytochemicals) is now available in capsule form. However, the studies linking lycopene to a reduced risk of certain forms of cancer have all been done on food and not on supplements. Therefore, I still recommend getting your lycopene from food if you can.

POSSIBLE BENEFITS

Cancer Fighter • A handful of studies have linked low blood serum levels of lycopene to an increased risk of certain forms of cancer. No one is certain how lycopene may offer protection against cancer; however, most researchers believe that its antioxidant properties may play a role.

- A study at the School of Public Health and the University of Illinois at Chicago showed a link between lycopene blood levels and cervical dysplasia, a precancerous condition in women.
- Bladder cancer is the most common malignant tumor of the urinary tract and is prevalent among fifty- to seventy-year-olds. Recent studies have shown a link between low blood levels of lycopene and an increased risk of bladder cancer.

- Pancreatic cancer, one of the most lethal forms of cancer, primarily affects people between the ages of fifty and eighty. There are 28,000 new cases of pancreatic cancer each year, and the disease is very difficult to treat. Researchers speculate that lycopene may offer some protection against pancreatic cancer based on a recent study that showed that people with the lowest levels of lycopene had the greatest risk of developing pancreatic tumors.

Magnesium

FACTS

As minerals go, magnesium is hardly a superstar—few people think about whether or not they're getting enough magnesium in the course of a day. And yet, as we age, magnesium may prove to be one of the most important anti-aging minerals.

Magnesium is essential for calcium and vitamin C metabolism and also plays a role in the metabolism of phosphorus, sodium, and potassium. This mineral is important for converting blood sugar into energy and is necessary for effective nerve and muscle functioning.

In recent years, magnesium has been touted as an essential mineral for heart health, and recent studies suggest that it may also play a role in helping to prevent diabetes, especially later in life.

Good sources of magnesium include nuts, unmilled grains, seeds, apricots, dried mustard, curry powder, dark leafy vegetables, and bananas.

THE RIGHT AMOUNT

The National Research Council recommends 250 to 350 milligrams daily for adults. Magnesium is available in most multivi-

tamin and mineral supplements and can also be purchased in
the form of magnesium oxide supplements (250 milligrams of
magnesium oxide = 150 milligrams of pure magnesium per
tablet).

Chelated magnesium (a more digestible form of the mineral) and calcium supplements (with half as much magnesium
and calcium) is an excellent source of both minerals.

People who drink heavily require extra magnesium.

**Caution: Excess magnesium (over 1000 milligrams daily)
can cause diarrhea. Over time, it can be toxic. Do not take a
magnesium supplement if you have kidney disease.**

POSSIBLE BENEFITS

Heart Disease   •   Epidemiological studies show that people
who live in regions with high levels of magnesium in the soil
and water have a lower rate of heart disease than the general
population. Many other studies have shown that people who
have heart attacks have a lower than normal level of magnesium in their body tissues. As far back as the 1950s, animal studies have shown that high doses of magnesium can actually
reverse atherosclerotic plaques. Other studies show that magnesium decreases blood pressure and improves the flow of blood to
the heart. It's logical to conclude that magnesium plays some
role in protecting against heart disease, although the precise
role is not known. Some researchers, however, believe that
magnesium works in conjunction with calcium to prevent fatal
arrhythmias, similar to calcium channel blockers.

In many hospitals, intravenous magnesium is routinely
given to patients after they have a heart attack. The effectiveness of this treatment is still under debate. Several studies have
shown that people who get intravenous magnesium after a heart
attack have a significantly better survival rate than those who
don't. However, a major U.S. study involving thousands of heart
attack patients did not support magnesium's use post–heart attack.

Improves Glucose Handling   •   As people age, they are likely
to develop insulin resistance, that is, they cannot use insulin ef-

ficiently to turn glucose into energy, thus blood glucose levels rise, which can lead to diabetes. According to a recent study at the University of Naples, magnesium supplements can improve glucose handling in older people with insulin resistance. Other studies have shown that magnesium supplements can reduce blood pressure and lower the risk of complications in patients who already have diabetes.

Melatonin

FACTS

Melatonin is a hormone secreted by the pineal gland in the brain during sleep. Melatonin is vital for the maintenance of normal body rhythms, especially the sleep–wake cycle, and appears to play a critical role in many other body functions. When I'm on the road, I use melatonin to help ease the symptoms of jet lag, when normal sleep patterns are disturbed by a disruption in the daylight–darkness pattern. Melatonin helps to normalize the body's circadian rhythm, which regulates sleep–wake cycles. Recently, melatonin has been successfully tested as a cure for insomnia.

The production of melatonin declines dramatically with age. Today, many researchers suspect that melatonin may be a natural anti-aging hormone.

THE RIGHT AMOUNT

Synthetic forms of melatonin are sold in natural food stores in tablet or capsule form in 3-milligram strength. A faster-acting sublingual tablet, which is placed under the tongue, is also available. Take 1 to 2 tablets or capsules about 1½ hours before bedtime. If using the sublingual form, take them 45 minutes before going to sleep. Occasional use preferred. (Do not drive or operate heavy machinery after taking melatonin.)

POSSIBLE BENEFITS

Longevity • In 1987, Walter Pierpaoli, M.D., Ph.D., and his colleagues at the Biancalana-Masera Foundation for the Aged in Ancona, Italy, showed that adding melatonin to the drinking water of mice during darkness prolonged the life span of the animals by more than 20 percent (about six months longer than average). The researchers speculated that melatonin may help reduce stress and improve the function of the immune system in animals and, perhaps, in humans. Other animal studies have shown that the removal of the pineal gland (which produces melatonin) can result in an acceleration of the aging process. In a review article published in *The International Journal of Neuroscience* (Vol. 52, 1990, pp. 85–92), psychiatrist Reuven Sandyk of the Department of Psychiatry of Albert Einstein College of Medicine in New York stated, "There is evidence from both experimental animal and human studies to suggest that decreased melatonin functions may accelerate the aging process and thus support the notion that melatonin may function as an anti-aging hormone."

Some researchers speculate that melatonin may be an antioxidant, that is, it prevents cellular damage associated with aging by thwarting the action of free radicals. Others feel that melatonin may slow down aging by controlling the timing of the release of certain hormones, proteins, and neurotransmitters (chemicals that help nerve cells communicate with each other).

Insomnia • Disruption in sleep cycles is a common ailment among older people, and many scientists have suggested that a reduction in melatonin may be responsible. In fact, recent studies show that melatonin may be a potent sleep aid. Researchers at Massachusetts Institute of Technology in Boston have shown that melatonin can induce sleep in young volunteers within 5 or 6 minutes. Volunteers given a placebo took 15 minutes or more to fall asleep. In addition, those taking the melatonin slept twice as long as those taking the placebo. Scientists hope that melatonin may prove to be a safe, nonaddicting sleep agent.

Breast Cancer • Several studies have linked a higher rate of breast cancer to both women and men who are in professions where they are exposed to low-frequency electronic magnetic fields (EMFs). Researchers were puzzled by this finding and were not certain how or even if EMFs played a role in cancer. However, one recent study showed that exposure to EMFs can reduce the pineal gland's ability to produce melatonin at night. Test tube studies have shown that melatonin can inhibit the growth of breast tumor cells; therefore, some researchers now suspect that low blood levels of melatonin may promote the growth of breast tumors. Although these findings are interesting, as of yet, scientists caution that the case of EMFs and melatonin is far from closed and much more research is needed.

Menadione (Vitamin K)

FACTS

When *Earl Mindell's Vitamin Bible* was first published in 1979, little was known about menadione, also called vitamin K, except that it was essential for the synthesis of proteins involved in proper blood clotting. Nearly two decades later, however, vitamin K is attracting the attention of researchers worldwide because of the possible role it may play in helping to prevent osteoporosis. In fact, at the U.S. Department of Agriculture's Human Nutrition Research Center at Tufts University, there is a special laboratory devoted to investigating the relationship between vitamin K and aging.

Vitamin K is formed by intestinal bacteria. It is also found in green leafy vegetables, alfalfa, egg yolks, safflower oil, soybean oil, kelp (seaweed), and fish liver oil.

THE RIGHT AMOUNT

The recommended daily allowance for vitamin K is 80 micrograms for men and 65 micrograms for women. I recommend taking a supplement of 50 to 100 micrograms daily. Do not exceed 500 micrograms daily. According to researchers at Tufts, older people may require higher levels of vitamin K due to a decreased rate of absorption.

People on long-term antibiotic regimens may develop a vitamin K deficiency.

Caution: People taking blood thinners should not take vitamin K unless under the supervision of a physician.

POSSIBLE BENEFITS

Osteoporosis • Several studies have shown that vitamin K supplements may help reduce the loss of calcium in urine, thus preventing the thinning of bones. For example, in one Dutch study presented at the New York Academy of Sciences special meeting on vitamins in 1991, researchers noted that a vitamin K supplement reduced urinary excretion of calcium in postmenopausal women and was particularly effective in stemming the loss of calcium among fast losers of calcium. Previous studies have linked a low level of vitamin K to an increased risk of fractures.

Milk Thistle

FACTS

Milk thistle preparations are popping up in natural food stores and are already extremely popular in the United States. Since ancient times, the seeds from this weed have been used to treat many different ailments including digestive disorders. However, today milk thistle is fast becoming known as the "liver herb."

Milk thistle contains silymarin, a compound that belongs to

the flavonoid family. Flavonoids are antioxidants and help protect cells from free radicals, unstable oxygen molecules that can cause dangerous mutations.

THE RIGHT AMOUNT

Milk thistle is available in capsules. Take 175 milligrams three times daily.

POSSIBLE BENEFITS

Liver Disease • The liver is the most complicated organ in the human body. It performs many vital tasks including the production of bile, which is necessary for the breakdown of fat and the storage of glycogen to fuel the muscles. The liver also produces other important substances such as clotting factors (so we don't bleed to death), blood proteins, and more than one thousand different enzymes. One of the liver's most critical roles is the detoxification of drugs and poisons, such as alcohol, which may be taken externally or produced internally. Injury to the liver can be life threatening. Inflammation of the liver is called *hepatitis* and can be caused by drug toxicity and viral infection. Many studies have shown that milk thistle has a strong therapeutic effect on the liver, protecting it from damage inflicted by toxins and disease. In fact, in Europe, milk thistle has been used as an effective treatment for viral hepatitis and cirrhosis of the liver (a condition often caused by alcohol abuse). Many people take milk thistle daily as a liver tonic to strengthen and protect this important organ.

Monounsaturated Fat

FACTS

Fat has become a dirty word lately, especially for people who are concerned about health and longevity, but eating monounsaturated fat may actually help you live longer. Studies show that in countries such as Italy and Greece, where the diet is rich in monounsaturated fat (mainly olive oil), the incidence of heart disease is a fraction of what it is in the United States.

There are three kinds of fats: saturated, polyunsaturated, and monounsaturated. The degree of saturation is determined by the number of hydrogen molecules: the more hydrogen molecules, the more saturated the fat. Saturated fat is believed to promote the formation of plaque, which can lead to atherosclerosis.

Olive, canola, and avocado oils are excellent sources of monounsaturated fat. Nuts such as almonds, peanuts, and walnuts are also rich in monounsaturates.

THE RIGHT AMOUNT

I believe that people should consume no more than 20 percent of their daily calories in the form of fat of any kind. (The American Heart Association recommends no more than 30 percent fat from daily calories, which I believe is too high. The late Nathan Pritikin and Dean Ornish, M.D., recommend no more than 10 percent, which I feel may be too difficult to adhere to.) Therefore, it's important to watch fat intake, even if it's "good" fat.

Use 1 to 2 tablespoons of olive or canola oil in your salad or cooking daily.

If you eat nuts, keep the portions small.

POSSIBLE BENEFITS

Heart Healthy • Although monounsaturated oil doesn't necessarily lower total blood cholesterol levels, it does raise the levels of high-density lipoproteins, or "good" cholesterol. High levels of high-density lipoproteins are associated with lower rates of heart disease.

Recently, Israeli researchers found that olive oil was less prone to oxidative damage than polyunsaturated oil. Oxidative damage of blood lipids is believed to be a major cause of atherosclerotic lesions that can lead to a heart attack or stroke. Olive oil in particular is also high in vitamin E, an antioxidant that helps prevent heart disease and cancer.

Diabetes • A handful of studies suggest that monounsaturated fat may be beneficial for diabetics.

Longevity • Other studies have linked consumption of monounsaturated foods—notably nuts—to a longer life span and a dramatically lower rate of heart attack. In fact, a major study of 26,000 members of the Seventh Day Adventist Church showed that those who ate almonds, peanuts, and walnuts at least six times a week had an average life span 7 years longer than the general population.

PERSONAL ADVICE

Keep in mind that fat in any form contains 9 calories per gram (as compared to 4 calories per gram for carbohydrates and protein). As beneficial as monounsaturated fats may be, a little goes along way.

Motherwort

FACTS

As its common name implies, motherwort has a long tradition of being used to treat problems of the female reproductive system. The Latin name for motherwort is *Lenonurus cardiaca*, and as that name implies, motherwort is also known as a heart healthy herb.

Motherwort contains compounds that can cause uterine contractions. For thousands of years, motherwort has been prescribed by herbal healers to bring on delayed menstruation or to speed up childbirth. However, today it is gaining popularity as a menopause aid.

THE RIGHT AMOUNT

Take 10 to 20 drops of motherwort in liquid up to three times daily, or drink 1 cup of tea.
Caution: Do not use this herb during pregnancy.

POSSIBLE BENEFITS

Heart • Motherwort is a mild sedative. It helps control palpitations and rapid heartbeat due to anxiety. It also temporarily lowers blood pressure. This herb is frequently used to treat anxiety related to the physiological changes that can occur during menopause.

Bloating • During menopause, women often retain water due to hormonal swings. This herb is a mild diuretic that can help relieve some of the discomfort due to bloating.

PERSONAL ADVICE

If you are experiencing rapid heartbeat or palpitations, check with your physician or natural healer. It could be a sign of a more serious problem.

Niacin (Vitamin B$_3$)

FACTS

If you have high cholesterol or have had a heart attack, this vitamin could save your life.

Niacin works with two other B vitamins, thiamine and riboflavin, in the metabolism of carbohydrates. It is also essential for providing energy for cell tissue growth. The body produces niacin from tryptophan, which is abundant in milk and eggs. Recent studies suggest that as people cut back on high-fat and high-cholesterol foods, such as milk and egg products, they may become deficient in niacin.

In recent years, niacin has gained fame as a potent cholesterol-lowering agent.

THE RIGHT AMOUNT

The recommended daily allowance for women is 15 milligrams and for men, 19 milligrams. High doses—the kind prescribed to cut cholesterol—can result in unpleasant side effects such as flushing and itching. If you are using niacin to lower cholesterol, I recommend the "no flush" niacin supplements with inositol hexanicotinate. Supplements are available in 50- to 1000-milligram-dose tablets or capsules. Usually, between 800 and 1200 milligrams daily are needed to lower cholesterol. However, you can reduce the niacin dose by taking it with chromium: take 100 milligrams of niacin with 600 micrograms of chromium daily.

Caution: High levels of niacin can interfere with the control of uric acid, bringing on attacks of gout in people who are prone to this disease. In addition, niacin may interfere with the body's ability to dispose of glucose and may promote liver abnormalities. Therefore, I recommend using niacin under the supervision of a physician. (Given the side effects of some of the other cholesterol-lowering drugs, niacin is relatively safe.)

POSSIBLE BENEFITS

Heart Disease • In 1975, the Coronary Drug Project, a major study, reported that niacin could dramatically reduce cholesterol levels and, even better, could cut the rate of second heart attacks by 30 percent. A 15-year follow-up study comparing niacin to clofibrate, another cholesterol-lowering drug, found that even though both agents lowered cholesterol, patients who had taken the niacin had significantly fewer heart-related deaths than those who had taken the clofibrate.

Other studies confirm that niacin can lower both cholesterol and triglycerides and can raise the level of high-density lipoproteins, or "good" cholesterol.

Cancer Fighter • There's some evidence that niacin may offer some protection against cancer. In a recent study, scientists at the University of Kentucky's Markey Center tested the effect of niacin deficiency on human and animal cells. Cells that were deprived of niacin began to show signs of malignant changes that could lead to cancer. More studies need to be done on the role of niacin in cancer.

Nitrosamine Blockers

FACTS

Nitrosamines are cancer-causing compounds that are formed during normal digestion. Nitrosamines can occur when nitrites, a commonly used food preservative, or nitrates, a naturally occurring chemical in food, combine with amino acids. Nitrosamines can destroy DNA, which can lead to cancerous changes in cells. Several years ago, researchers at Cornell University reported that certain foods, such as tomatoes, green peppers, strawberries, pineapples, and carrots, can prevent the formation of these troublesome nitrosamines. Initially, scientists believed that vitamin C was the primary nitrosamine blocker in these foods. However, in a recent article in *Agriculture and Food Chemistry,* Cornell University food scientists reported the discovery of two other compounds in tomatoes—*p*-courmaric acid and chlorogenic acids—that appear to be potent nitrosamine blockers. This discovery has led scientists to believe that there are probably other nitrosamine blockers in fruits and vegetables that have yet to be identified.

You can't get these compounds in a pill or capsule—you must eat fruits and vegetables. Cooking doesn't destroy these compounds, and they are also present in juice.

The Right Amount

There's no recommended daily allowance for nitrosamine blockers. Eat a wide variety of fruits and vegetables daily. I make it a point to eat a tomato or drink a glass of tomato juice daily.

Possible Benefits

Cancer Fighter • Researchers at Cornell University tested tomato juice on volunteers. After drinking the juice, the volunteers produced fewer cancer-causing nitrosamines. Although more studies need to be done, there is evidence that eating foods rich in nitrosamine blockers may help to prevent cancer.

Personal Advice

Nitrites are added to cured meats such as bacon and hot dogs to prevent botulism and as a coloring agent. Try to buy nitrite-free products, which are available at many supermarkets and meat markets.

Nucleic Acids (DNA and RNA)

Facts

DNA (deoxyribonucleic acid) and RNA (ribonucleic acid) are present in the nucleus of every cell in the body and are essential for the production of new cells, cell repair, and cell metabolism. As we age, cells begin to wear out and eventually die. When we're young, we grow new cells very quickly, but as we age, we replenish cells more slowly. Internally, our body systems begin to slow down, and externally, we begin to show signs of wear and tear. Some researchers believe that aging may be a result of a decline in the level or effectiveness of these important nucleic acids. The theory goes, if we replenish the lost nucleic acids, we may be able to halt or even reverse the aging process.

Good food sources of nucleic acids include Portuguese sardines (water packed), salmon, wheat germ, asparagus, mushrooms, and spinach. Nucleic acids are also available in supplement form at natural food stores.

THE RIGHT AMOUNT

Combinations of DNA and RNA are sold in tablet form at natural food stores. Take 1 to 3 tablets (up to 1500 milligrams) daily. I have been doing so for over thirty years.

Caution: Drink at least 8 glasses of fluid daily if you are taking nucleic acids in supplement form or are eating a diet rich in nucleic acids. RNA can raise uric acid levels, which may trigger gout in susceptible people. If you have a tendency to develop gout, do not take nucleic acids.

POSSIBLE BENEFITS

Longevity • A handful of studies suggest that nucleic acids may increase the life span of animals. For example, in one study reported in *The Journal of the American Geriatrics Society* almost two decades ago, five laboratory rats were given weekly injections of DNA and RNA, and five were untreated. The untreated mice died within 900 days; however, the treated mice lived between 1600 to 2250 days. Researchers also noted that the mice given nucleic acids looked healthier and were more alert than the other mice. More studies need to be done to confirm whether nucleic acids are truly a "fountain of youth."

There is anecdotal evidence, however, that nucleic acids may have a dramatic effect on humans. In his book, *Nucleic Acid Therapy in Aging and Degenerative Disease*, Benjamin Frank, M.D., reports on his experiences treating patients with nucleic acid therapy. Based on Dr. Frank's observations, patients given nucleic acid supplements showed a marked improvement in the color and texture of their skin, a reduction in age spots, and an increase in energy level.

Oat Bran

FACTS

Oat bran contains a compound called beta-glucan, a potent cholesterol-lowering agent. Beta-glucan is a form of soluble fiber.

Good sources of oat bran include oat bran cereal and high-fiber oatmeal. Instant oatmeal (the kind that cooks in the bowl) usually has less oat bran than regular oatmeal.

THE RIGHT AMOUNT

A bowl of oatmeal and an oat bran muffin daily can help reduce a high cholesterol level and keep normal cholesterol in check.

POSSIBLE BENEFITS

Heart Disease • There have been numerous studies documenting oat bran's ability to lower cholesterol. When combined with a normal low-fat diet, about 2 ounces of oats daily can reduce cholesterol by 5 to 10 percent. Oat bran can also lower low-density lipoproteins, the "bad" cholesterol, and can raise high-density lipoproteins, the "good" cholesterol.

Diabetes • Researchers at the University of Kentucky have found that oat bran can help improve glucose and blood lipid levels in diabetics, helping diabetics reduce or eliminate their need for insulin.

Octacosanol

FACTS

Octacosanol is a natural substance present in small amounts in many vegetable oils. A popular commercially marketed form of octacosanol is made from wheat germ oil. Proponents of octacosanol contend that it is a treasure trove of phytochemicals that can increase energy, improve oxygen utilization, and even prevent heart disease. Octacosanol is an excellent source of another member of the anti-aging hot 100: vitamin E.

Good food sources of octacosanol include wheat germ, whole grains, and alfalfa.

THE RIGHT AMOUNT

Supplements of 1000 to 6000 micrograms per tablet are available at natural food stores. Take one daily.

POSSIBLE BENEFITS

Improves Stamina • Studies suggest that octacosanol may improve exercise performance in animals and humans. Octacosanol is believed to reduce oxygen debt, that is, it helps the body utilize oxygen more efficiently during times of stress. Therefore, if you use octacosanol, you're less likely to be huffing and puffing after a strenuous workout.

Heart Disease • Octacosanol contains plant sterols, compounds that have been shown to reduce cholesterol levels in animal and human studies. However, the high vitamin E content of octacosanol may also play a role in reducing cholesterol by preventing the oxidation of low-density lipoproteins, or "bad" cholesterol, which can lead to the clogging of important arteries.

Omega-3 Fatty Acids

FACTS

In the 1970s, scientists noticed an interesting phenomenon: although Eskimos consumed large amounts of fat daily, they had an exceptionally low rate of heart disease and cancer. But unlike Americans who also ate lots of fat—notably from meat and dairy—the predominant fat in the Eskimo diet was in the form of omega-3 fatty acids. Omega-3 is found primarily in marine plant life called *phytoplankton,* which is eaten by fatty fish, a mainstay of the Eskimo diet. On land, omega-3 is present in some plant food including flaxseed and purslane, a plant that is used in salads.

Since the 1970s, there have been hundreds of studies performed worldwide on omega-3 fatty acids. These studies have shown that omega-3 does indeed offer protection against heart disease and possibly many other ailments.

Omega-3 contains two polyunsaturated fats: decosahexaenioc acid and eicosapentaenoic acid.

Good sources include fish such as salmon, mackerel, albacore tuna, halibut, and sardines.

THE RIGHT AMOUNT

According to the National Heart and Lung Institute, eating as little as 1 gram of omega-3 fatty acids daily may reduce the risk of cardiovascular disease by as much as 40 percent. Omega-3 fatty acids are available in capsule form. Take 3 to 6 capsules daily.

Super eicosapentaenoic acid—a more concentrated form—is also available. Take three capsules daily.

Flaxseed oil capsules are another source of omega-3 fatty acids. Take 1 or 2 capsules (1000 milligrams) daily with meals.

However, fatty fish is the best source of omega-3 fatty acids. In fact, studies suggest that the whole fish may be more effective than simply taking an oil supplement.

Caution: Do not take omega-3 supplements if you are already taking a blood thinner (such as coumadin or heparin) or using aspirin daily without first consulting with your physician. Excessive amounts of omega-3 fatty acids may cause bleeding, which can result in hemorraghic stroke.

POSSIBLE BENEFITS

Heart Disease   •   Epidemiological studies document a lower rate of coronary artery disease among fish eaters among Greenland's Eskimo population and the Japanese.

Omega-3 fatty acids appear to have several positive effects on cardiovascular health. Omega-3 fatty acids are blood thinners and may help prevent the formation of blood clots that can lead to a heart attack. A recent study of fifteen thousand people in four communities in the United States demonstrated that an increased intake of fatty fish can make a positive difference in terms of cardiovascular health. In this study, researchers compared the level of clotting factors (proteins found in the blood that can contribute to the formation of clots) to the amount of fatty fish in people's diet. Those who ate even one additional daily serving of fish had lower levels of three clotting factors that have been implicated in the development of coronary artery disease. Those with the highest levels of omega-3 fatty acid intake had higher levels of a fourth protein, protein C, a natural anticoagulant.

Several studies have shown that omega-3 fatty acids can lower total cholesterol and triglycerides in people who also cut back on saturated fat. In a Danish study, pathologists who autopsied fatty abdominal tissue and coronary arteries of forty deceased people found a direct correlation between the amount of omega-3 fatty acids in the tissue and the degree of narrowing of the coronary arteries due to atherosclerosis. In other words, omega-3 fatty acids appear to prevent the formation of atherosclerotic plaque, which can hamper the flow of blood to the heart.

A recent animal study performed at Australia's Commonwealth Scientific and Industrial Research Organization in Adelaide investigated the effects of dietary fat on susceptibility to ventricular fibrillation, a potentially lethal heart arrhythmia. (Ventricular fibrillation may be responsible for as many as 250,000 deaths in the United States annually.) According to the study, animals who were fed fish oil were better able to withstand induced heart arrhythmias than animals fed sunflower oil. The researchers concluded that omega-3 fatty acids may help prevent heart arrhythmias in humans.

Stroke • A long-term Dutch study shows men who consumed more than 20 grams (about 0.67 ounce) of fish per day had a lower risk of stroke than those who ate less fish. This is believed to be the first reported finding between higher fish consumption and lower stroke risk.

Cancer Fighter • In numerous animal studies, omega-3 fatty acids have delayed the onset of tumors and decreased both the rate of growth, size, and number of tumors in animals in which cancer was induced. Interestingly enough, in similar studies, other forms of fat typically increased tumor growth.

Arthritis • Omega-3 fatty acids have an anti-inflammatory action in the human body, that is, they alter the biological pathways that trigger inflammation, which is responsible for the pain and stiffness of arthritis and other related conditions. In several studies, patients with rheumatoid arthritis reported a decrease in symptoms after taking omega-3 fatty acid supplements in addition to their nonsteroid antirheumatic drugs.

Diabetes • In a Dutch study of 175 older people (sixty-four to eighty-seven) for 3 years, those who ate fish were least likely to develop glucose intolerance, a common problem among older adults that can lead to diabetes.

Papain

FACTS

If you find yourself popping more and more antacids, you're not alone. As we age, our digestive system gets less efficient. As a result, indigestion is a common malady among people over fifty. Natural compounds such as papain, which is derived from papaya, may help to quiet an angry gut. Papain contains two enzymes, papain and prolase, which help to break down protein.

THE RIGHT AMOUNT

Chewable papaya supplements are sold in natural food stores. Chew 1 to 3 tablets ½ hour before eating.

POSSIBLE BENEFITS

Digestive Aid • In older people, indigestion is often due to the inability of the body to produce enough hydrochloric acid to break down food effectively. Although there has been little scientific research in this area, anecdotal evidence suggests that papain supplements may help improve digestion and reduce the need for antacids.

PERSONAL ADVICE

If you're experiencing a great deal of gas or bloating, although it's probably simple indigestion, it could be a symptom of another underlying problem. Check with your physician before self-medicating.

Pectin

FACTS

Everyone has heard that an apple a day will keep the doctor away. However, not everyone knows that pectin may be the reason why apples are so healthful. Pectin is a form of soluble fiber found in fruits and vegetables. Recent studies suggest that pectin may be a potent force against both cancer and heart disease.

Good food sources of pectin include apples, bananas, the pulpy portion of grapefruit, dried beans, and root vegetables.

THE RIGHT AMOUNT

Try to eat some pectin-rich foods daily. If you have high cholesterol, consider taking pectin capsules, which are available at
most natural food stores. Take 1 or 2 capsules after each meal.
Pectin powder is also sold in natural food stores; sprinkle ½
ounce of pectin powder in your food. It is flavorless and adds
body to yogurt, puddings, or fruit salads.

POSSIBLE BENEFITS

Heart Disease • Several forms of pectin appear to lower
blood cholesterol levels. Researchers at the University of
Florida gave twenty-seven people with high cholesterol either 3
tablespoons of powdered grapefruit pectin daily or a placebo.
After 16 weeks, the group taking the pectin showed a 7.6 percent reduction in cholesterol and a 10.8 percent reduction in
low-density lipoproteins, or "bad" cholesterol. The group taking
the placebo showed no change. Although powdered grapefruit
pectin is more potent than plain grapefruit, eating one or two
whole grapefruits daily—not just the segments, but the pulpy
portion between the segments—would probably also significantly lower cholesterol (in combination with a low-fat diet).

Carrot, which contains calcium pectate, also appears to be
a cholesterol buster. In fact, according to the U.S. Department
of Agriculture, eating two carrots a day may reduce total cholesterol levels by as much as 20 percent.

Eating two apples a day may keep the cardiologist away. A
recent study showed that people who ate two apples daily can
reduce total cholesterol by as much as 16 percent.

Cancer Fighter • Researchers at the University of Texas
Health Science Center in San Antonio recently discovered that
fiber may help to prevent colon cancer. The researchers fed laboratory rats a carcinogenic agent that predisposed them to develop colon cancer. One group of rats was fed a high-pectin
diet, the other group was fed a normal diet. After 24 weeks, the
group on the high-pectin diet had a significantly lower rate of
colon cancer than those fed the regular diet. (In addition, the

rats on the high-pectin diet had a 30 percent drop in cholesterol.) The pectin performed two roles: it increased the rate at which food passed through the gastrointestinal tract, which reduced the rat's exposure to carcinogens. Second, it bound with digestive bile, a derivative of cholesterol, thus reducing blood cholesterol levels.

Phytic Acid

FACTS

In the 1970s, researcher Denis Burkit published a now-famous study in which he showed that in third world countries where people ate a diet rich in plant foods, the rate of various forms of cancer was significantly lower than in the West. Dr. Burkit attributed the reduced rate of cancer to a higher intake of fiber, and soon Americans were loading up on bran and other sources of fiber. However, some researchers speculate that although fiber may be beneficial, the real hero may be phytic acid, a major ingredient in grains, nuts, and legumes (dried beans such as soybeans and lentils).

Phytic acid is an antioxidant; it protects cells against oxidative damage from free radicals or unstable oxygen molecules, which can cause mutations in DNA. Phytic acid is also a chelator, which means that it binds easily to metal, particularly iron. In the presence of oxygen, iron can create free radicals that attack DNA. Phytic acid can prevent this damage from occurring by binding with the iron, thus keeping it away from oxygen.

THE RIGHT AMOUNT

There is no recommended daily allowance for phytic acid. I recommend eating a diet rich in grains and legumes. Although nuts are an excellent source of phytic acid, they tend to be high in fat, so eat them sparingly.

POSSIBLE BENEFITS

Cancer Fighter   •   In several animal studies, phytic acid has been shown to inhibit the growth of tumors, especially in the colon. In one review of phytic acid published in *Free Radical Biology and Medicine* (Vol. 8, 1990) researchers noted that in populations where people eat high quantities of red meat, which is rich in iron, "the simultaneous presence of phytate may act to suppress iron-driven steps in carcinogenesis."

Potassium

FACTS

More than sixty million American adults have high blood pressure, which is a leading cause of heart attack and stroke. (High pressure is characterized by a systolic pressure over 140, and a diastolic pressure over 90.) The older you are, the greater the risk of developing this potentially lethal disease. There is strong evidence that dietary potassium intake may help to prevent high blood pressure and may even be used to enhance the effect of antihypertensive medications.

Potassium is an essential mineral that assists in muscle contraction and works with sodium to maintain the fluid and electrolyte balance in body cells. Nerve and muscle function may suffer when the sodium–potassium balance is off. Potassium is also critical to maintaining a normal heartbeat. In cases of severe potassium deficiency, the heart can develop a dangerous arrhythmia or irregular beat.

Potassium is found in fruits and vegetables and dairy products. Good sources include bananas, oranges, cantaloupe, dried apricots, squash, and plain low-fat yogurt.

THE RIGHT AMOUNT

The Food and Nutrition Board of the National Academy of Sciences has estimated the minimum requirement for potassium for adults to be 2000 milligrams daily. Potassium is available in most high-potency multivitamin and multimineral preparations. Excess amounts (over 18 grams) can be toxic. (Ninety milligrams per tablet or capsule is the maximum dosage allowed by law. A banana contains 560 milligrams of potassium.)

If you consume large quantities of coffee, are taking diuretics, have severe diarrhea and/or vomiting, or have hypoglycemia (low blood sugar), you may be deficient in this mineral. People on very low calorie weight-loss diets may also have a potassium deficiency.

Caution: People with kidney disease should not take potassium supplement or consume foods high in potassium.

POSSIBLE BENEFITS

Lowers Blood Pressure   •   A recent Italian study reported in *The Annals of Internal Medicine* (115, 1991: 753–759) underscored the importance of eating a diet rich in potassium, especially if you have high blood pressure. Fifty-four patients with controlled hypertension were randomly assigned to one of two groups. One group was given advice aimed at increasing potassium intake through diet; the other remained on their usual diet. Potassium intake among both groups was checked monthly by referring to patient food dairies and urinary potassium excretion. At the end of the year, the group on the high-potassium diet found that they needed far less medicine to control their blood pressure than the group not eating potassium-rich foods. The researchers concluded "increasing the dietary potassium intake from natural foods is a feasible and effective measure to reduce antihypertensive drug treatment."

PERSONAL ADVICE

If you're taking medication for high blood pressure, don't discontinue it, but work with your physician to see if you can decrease your need for medication by increasing your potassium intake. Eating a banana and a baked potato daily can increase your potassium intake by 1200 milligrams.

Propolis

FACTS

Propolis is a by-product of honey. It is a resinous material made from leaf parts and tree bark that is used by honeybees to cement together their hives. For thousands of years, honey and its related products have been valued for their medicinal properties. Hippocrates used propolis to treat sores and ulcers. Nicholas Culpepper (1616–1654)—perhaps the most famous herbalist of all time—recommended propolis to be used externally on wounds. Modern herbalists use propolis to ease cold symptoms and soothe a sore throat. Recently, scientists worldwide have begun to recognize that propolis may not only be an effective treatment for minor ailments, but may help to prevent a very major one: cancer.

THE RIGHT AMOUNT

Propolis is available in many different forms. Honey is rich in propolis. Pure propolis is available in capsule form at natural food stores. Take 500-milligram capsules up to three times daily.

Propolis salve may be used externally on sores. Propolis lozenges (which have a pleasant, sweet taste) are good for a sore throat.

POSSIBLE BENEFITS

Cancer Fighter • For decades, proponents of natural foods have touted propolis for its anticancer properties. Recently, serious researchers have investigated these claims. Researchers at the American Health Foundation in Valhalla, New York, tested caffeic acid esters, a compound found in propolis, for potential use against cancer. In the study, rats were fed a potent carcinogen. Some of the rats were also fed caffeic acid esters from propolis. After 9 weeks, the rats given the propolis compounds showed significantly less precancerous changes in colon cells than the rats not fed the propolis. Based on this and similar studies, it appears as if propolis can inhibit the growth of cancerous cells in the colon. Other studies are needed to determine whether propolis is useful against other forms of cancer.

Anti-inflammatory • Propolis may be similar to aspirin in that it also blocks the enzymes that produce prostaglandins, natural hormonelike substances that can cause pain, fever, and inflammation.

Antiviral • Propolis is rich in bioflavonoids, substances that appear to help protect against viral invasion. Viruses are encased in a protective protein coat. Researchers believe that the flavonoids in propolis may inhibit an enzyme in the body that strips viruses of their protective coating, thus allowing the infection to spread to other cells. As people age and their immune system weakens, propolis may give the immune system a much-needed boost against common viruses that can cause colds and flu.

Prevents Gum Disease • Periodontal problems are common from middle age on. Very often, as people age, the gum line begins to recede, causing inflammation, bleeding, and infection. This can lead to the weakening of the bone structure in the mouth, which can result in tooth loss. Some researchers believe that the flavonoids in propolis not only reduce inflammation, but also strengthen the blood vessels in the gums, making them less prone to injury.

Protease Inhibitors

FACTS

Protease inhibitors are compounds that inhibit the action of certain enzymes that promote tumor growth. The National Cancer Institute is investigating protease inhibitors for their potential anticancer properties.

Protease inhibitors are abundant in legumes (soy beans in particular and other dried beans) and whole grains.

THE RIGHT AMOUNT

There is no recommended daily allowance for protease inhibitors. I recommend eating at least one food daily that contains protease inhibitors.

POSSIBLE BENEFITS

Cancer Fighter • Several animal studies have shown that protease inhibitors can inhibit the growth of cancer. For example, soybeans contain a unique protease inhibitor: the Bowman–Birk inhibitor (BBI), which has been shown to stop the spread of many different forms of cancer. For example, in rats fed a carcinogen known to induce colon cancer, adding BBI concentrate to their diet suppressed the formation of tumors in 100 percent of the animals. In another study of mice fed a carcinogen known to induce liver cancer, BBI suppressed the formation of tumors by 71 percent. The National Cancer Institute is now conducting human cancer prevention trials using BBI in people at high risk of developing cancer.

Psyllium Seed

FACTS

Ground psyllium seed is a popular cure for constipation, a problem that seems to be a common ailment among the older population. For years, doctors have recommended psyllium as a natural way to regulate bowel function in people with digestive disorders such as irritable bowel syndrome and chronic constipation.

In addition, psyllium is a highly effective and safe cholesterol-lowering agent.

THE RIGHT AMOUNT

I recommend a teaspoon to a tablespoon of psyllium daily in juice or water. Psyllium is sold in powder form in drug stores and natural food stores. In fact, psyllium is the active ingredient in over-the-counter medications such as Metamucil and Fibercon. Some psyllium products contains other herbs, including slippery elm bark and acidophilus, which can help ease some of the gas and bloating that can occur when you aren't used to psyllium. Check them out at your local natural food store.

Caution: Although it is rare, psyllium can cause allergic reactions in some sensitive individuals. If you are sensitive, talk to your physician before using psyllium. In addition, to prevent gas, drink 6 to 8 glasses of water daily.

POSSIBLE BENEFITS

Heart Disease • Several studies show that psyllium can lower blood cholesterol from high levels to safer levels. In one study, twenty-six men with cholesterol levels over 240 milligrams per deciliter were divided into two groups. (The range was 180 to 314 milligrams per deciliter.) One group was given 1 packet of Metamucil (3.4 grams) three times daily in water before each meal. At the end of 8 weeks, the average cholesterol level in the treatment group dropped to 211 milligrams per deciliter. The level of low-density lipoproteins, or "bad" cholesterol, also dropped substantially.

In another study by fiber expert James W. Anderson of the University of Kentucky Medical Service, forty-four people with elevated cholesterol levels were given either psyllium flake cereal or wheat bran flake cereal daily for 6 weeks. The results: the group eating the psyllium flake cereal had an average 12 percent drop in cholesterol, but the group eating the wheat bran had no change.

Quercetin

FACTS

Quercetin is a bioflavonoid, a group of compounds found in fruits and vegetables. Many bioflavonoids are now being studied for their ability to prevent disease.

Quercetin, an antioxidant, also may have antiviral properties when combined with vitamin C. Several studies suggest that quercetin may be a potent cancer fighter.

The best food sources of quercetin are yellow and red onions and shallots. High levels are also found in broccoli and zucchini.

THE RIGHT AMOUNT

There is no recommended daily allowance for quercetin. In addition, quercetin is also available in supplement form, often in combination with other bioflavonoids or antioxidants. The usual dose is 250 milligrams one or two times daily.

POSSIBLE BENEFITS

Cancer Fighter • In many studies, quercetin has been shown to block the action of a variety of natural and synthetic initiators or promoters of cancer cell development. In addition, quercetin appears to inhibit the growth of human tumor cells containing binding sites for type II estrogen, which may be responsible for some forms of cancer, including breast cancer.

Population studies have shown that people who eat a diet rich in onions and other allium vegetables have substantially lower rates of gastrointestinal cancers than people who don't. Scientists are not precisely sure why onion protects against cancer—they do contain many potentially beneficial phytochemicals—but high levels of quercetin may be a major factor.

Anti-allergy   •   An allergy is an inflammatory condition triggered by an allergen, any substance—either natural or synthetic—that causes an allergic antibody reaction in the body. In an allergic antibody reaction, the immune system mistakenly identifies a harmless substance as a dangerous invader and begins to produce chemicals against it, including histamine. Histamine is responsible for sneezing, an itchy nose, watery eyes, and some of the other unpleasant allergic symptoms. Studies show that quercetin prevents the release of histamine, thus inhibiting the allergic response. Interestingly enough, several other bioflavonoidlike substances are marketed as allergy medications. Quercetin may also be useful against asthma.

Reishi Mushroom

FACTS

Aging takes its toll on the immune system. As people age, their immune systems become less effective at identifying foreign agents and fighting against viruses and bacteria. As a result, they are more vulnerable to cancer, infections, and other related problems. Reishi mushroom, known for its powerful immune-stimulating properties, is one of the most revered foods in Japan.

THE RIGHT AMOUNT

Reishi is available as capsules at natural food stores. Take 1 capsule up to three times daily.

POSSIBLE BENEFITS

Immune Booster • Studies show that compounds found in reishi mushrooms can increase the activity of two types of immune cells that are necessary to fight against potentially troublesome organisms.

Cancer Fighter • Compounds found in reishi mushrooms inhibited the growth of tumors in laboratory mice, which suggests that they may play a similar role in humans.

Heart Disease • Studies show that reishi mushrooms can lower cholesterol and reduce blood pressure.

Resveratrol

FACTS

For centuries, people have been drinking to each other's good health over an alcoholic beverage. And since biblical times, alcohol, especially wine, has been used as a traditional medicine for a wide range of ailments. In recent years, scientists have noticed that moderate drinkers tend to live longer than teetotalers. In fact, in countries where a glass of wine or two is a routine part of a meal, such as France and Italy, the incidence of heart disease is much lower than in countries where wine is not consumed in such great volume. Puzzled as to why wine drinkers fared so much better than non–wine drinkers, scientists began to examine the chemistry of wine to see what, if anything, could be offering its beneficial effects. Japanese researchers recently identified an antifungal compound in grape skins called *resveratrol* that lowers the fat content in the livers of rats, thus lowering overall cholesterol. Many scientists believe that resveratrol may have the same effect on humans, which is why a drink or two of wine a day may keep the cardiologist away.

THE RIGHT AMOUNT

Drink 1 or 2 glasses of wine several times a week. If you are taking any medication, check with your physician before drinking any alcoholic beverage. Nonalcoholic wine is also available.

Caution: Too much wine counteracts any of its potential benefits. People who drink more than 1 or 2 glasses of wine per day are putting themselves at risk for developing cardiovascular and liver disease as well as other health problems. If you have a drinking problem, no amount of wine is safe for you.

POSSIBLE BENEFITS

Heart Healthy • Several major studies have confirmed that alcohol in general, and wine in particular, appears to protect against heart disease. A glass or two of wine can lower your blood pressure. Researchers recently discovered that resveratrol and other chemicals in wine are vasodilators, that is, they relax the blood vessels, allowing the blood to flow more easily.

Starting in 1978, a group of researchers at Kaiser Permanente Medical Center in Oakland, California, began a study to determine the effect of alcohol on coronary artery disease. The team collected information on 81,825 men and women. Over the next 10 years, the researchers monitored this group for deaths due to heart disease. The results: those who regularly drank alcoholic beverages had a lower rate of death from coronary artery disease, but those who drank wine had the lowest rate of all.

In yet other studies sponsored by the American Heart Association, people who consumed alcoholic beverages, especially wine, had up to 49 percent reduction in heart disease versus those who abstained.

Not only does alcohol appear to cut total cholesterol, but it also raises the rate of beneficial high-density lipoproteins (HDLs), or "good" cholesterol. People who drank at least 1 glass of wine daily have been found to have higher levels of HDL than non–wine drinkers. This is true for both men and women. In fact, for women, just 1 glass of wine daily is all it takes to raise HDLs; men require 2 glasses.

Riboflavin (Vitamin B$_2$)

FACTS

The primary function of this B vitamin is to work with other substances to metabolize carbohydrates, fats, and proteins for energy.

Riboflavin may also protect against certain forms of cancer and oxidative damage by free radicals.

People over fifty-five are at risk of developing a riboflavin deficiency, especially if they do not eat a well-rounded diet and do not take a vitamin supplement.

Good sources of riboflavin include no-fat or low-fat dairy products, eggs, and leafy vegetables. (Liver is also an excellent source of riboflavin. However, I don't recommend eating liver due to its high-cholesterol, high-fat content. Toxins—natural and synthetic—are also concentrated in liver.)

THE RIGHT AMOUNT

The recommended daily allowance (RDA) for riboflavin is 1.2 to 1.7 milligrams for adults. Riboflavin is included in most multivitamin supplements as well as in B-complex supplements. The usual dose is 100 to 300 milligrams.

Women who take estrogen need to take a B$_2$ supplement.

Riboflavin works best with vitamins B$_6$ and C and niacin.

POSSIBLE BENEFITS

Antioxidant • Riboflavin has antioxidant properties. It also works with the enzyme glutathione reductase to maintain glutathione, which fights against free radical damage. A particularly important role of riboflavin is to protect against oxidative damage during exercise when the demand for oxygen by the body increases.

Cancer Fighter • Low levels of this B vitamin may increase the risk of developing cancer of the esophagus, especially for people who chew tobacco or drink alcoholic beverages.

Healthy Eyes • Riboflavin can help to prevent damage to the cornea of the eye, which can result in cataracts.

Boosts Immunity • Riboflavin deficiency can decrease the number of T cells, an important component of the immune system. Low levels of T cells may increase the risk of developing cancer and other diseases.

For Active Women • Studies show that active older women may require higher levels of riboflavin than the RDA. Researchers at Cornell University recently studied the effect of riboflavin levels on exercise in women ages sixty to seventy. For 8 weeks, these women exercised for up to 25 minutes daily on a stationary bicycle. Half the group was given the RDA for riboflavin, the other half was given 150 percent of the RDA. Blood levels of B_2 dropped in the women who were given only the RDA. Researchers concluded that older women who exercise regularly may need extra riboflavin.

Saw Palmetto

FACTS

Native Americans ate the berries of the saw palmetto plant by the handful. Known by the botanical name *Serenoa repens*, naturopaths and herbalists in the United States and Europe have long used saw palmetto berries to treat problems of the genitourinary tract in both sexes. In fact, saw palmetto is a folk remedy for so-called honeymoon cystitis, a condition caused by too much sexual activity. This herb was also touted as an aphrodisiac. Today, in Germany, extract of saw palmetto is a leading treatment for benign prostate hypertrophy (enlarged prostate) and is reputed to be so successful that American doctors are taking a second look at this "archaic" medicine.

THE RIGHT AMOUNT

Saw palmetto is available in extract or capsule form at most health food stores and herb shops. Mix 30 to 60 drops in liquid daily, or take 1 to 3 capsules.

POSSIBLE BENEFITS

Prostate • In men, the prostate gland is a walnut-size organ surrounding the urethra, which is located at the neck of the bladder. By age fifty, most men develop a slightly enlarged prostate, a benign condition that can result in excessive urination, especially at night, or difficulty in passing urine. Benign prostate hypertrophy is believed to be caused by an excess buildup of testosterone, the male hormone, in the prostate. Excess testosterone is converted into dihydrotestosterone, a more potent form of the hormone that can promote cell growth, thus leading to the enlargement. Excess levels of testosterone are also believed to be linked to cancer of the prostate. Several scientific studies have shown that saw palmetto extracts can alter the biological pathways that lead to the conversion of testosterone to dihydrotestosterone. In addition, by preventing the more potent testosterone from binding to receptor sites on the cells, it may help rid the body of this potentially dangerous hormone.

Saw palmetto may not only help to prevent enlargement of the prostate, but has proven to be an effective treatment for this condition. In a 1984 study published in *The British Journal of Pharmacology*, 110 patients suffering from enlarged prostate were either given saw palmetto extract or a placebo for 30 days. Patients on saw palmetto experienced a significant reduction in symptoms, such as fewer nighttime urinations (down by 45 percent) and improved urine flow. Those on the placebo showed little change in their condition.

PERSONAL ADVICE

If you have discomfort or difficulty with urination or pass blood with your urine, check with your physician. Don't self-diagnose. However, if your physician confirms that you have benign prostate hypertrophy, try using saw palmetto to see if it helps. If you don't see any improvement within a month or so, talk to your physician about medication. Proscar, a relatively new drug, has been quite effective in treating an enlarged prostate. However, Proscar is quite expensive and may run up to several hundred dollars a year; saw palmetto extract costs a lot less and, in some cases, may work just as well.

Schizandra

FACTS

This highly prized Chinese herb is fast becoming a best-seller in the United States because of its reputation as a longevity herb and aphrodisiac. Since ancient times, schizandra has been favored among the wealthy Chinese. Until recently, this herb has been rare and expensive, but today it is widely available in China and the United States. Herbal healers have used schizandra to treat lung disorders, and recent studies show that extracts from this herb are effective against the bacteria that causes tuberculosis.

Similar to ginseng, schizandra is also believed to increase stamina and relieve fatigue. It is also used to treat stress and depression. According to one study, polo horses given schizandra performed better and showed better physiological responses to stress after taking the herb.

THE RIGHT AMOUNT

Schizandra is available in capsules at natural food stores. Take 1 to 3 capsules daily.

POSSIBLE BENEFITS

Liver • Animal studies have shown that this herb can help protect the liver from toxins, thus helping to preserve this vital organ.

Aphrodisiac • In China, schizandra is highly regarded as an aphrodisiac for both sexes. According to Ron Teeguarden, author of *Chinese Tonic Herbs*, "it relieves fatigue and is quite famous for increasing the sexual staying power in men." Teeguarden notes schizandra does no less for women, adding that it is reputed to cause "the female genitals to feel warm, healthy and extremely sensitive."

Seaweed

FACTS

Seaweed, also known as algae, is a primitive, plantlike organism that grows in the sea. Although seaweed is still considered exotic fare in the United States, it is a dietary mainstay in Japan.

Dietary seaweed is sold in the United States in Asian and natural food stores. There are several varieties of seaweed, or algae, differentiated by their color. Nori, a red seaweed, is used to wrap sushi. Popular forms of brown seaweed include kelp, wakame, arme, and kombu.

Traditional Chinese healers have used hot water extracts of seaweed to treat cancer. Not surprisingly, recent studies show that compounds in seaweed may protect against cancer.

THE RIGHT AMOUNT

There's no recommended daily allowance or study that specifies the correct amount of seaweed needed to prevent cancer. However, in Japan, where the cancer rate is a fraction of that in the United States, most people eat some form of seaweed daily. In fact, the estimated per capital intake of seaweed in Japan ranges from 4.9 to 7.3 grams daily (that's roughly ¼ ounce).

POSSIBLE BENEFITS

Cancer Fighter • Japanese scientists isolated several polysaccharides, potentially anticarcinogenic compounds, in seaweed. Fucoidin, one of these compounds, may prove to be a potent cancer fighter. Several studies show that these compounds in seaweed may have a dramatic impact on cancer. In one study, laboratory mice were injected with cancer cells. One group of mice received an extract from marine algae, the other group was given water without the extract. The life span of the treated mice was 37 percent longer than that of the control animals. Researchers speculate that the seaweed may somehow boost the body's immunological defenses against tumor growth. However, test tube studies also show that seaweed extract can prevent or slow down the growth of cancer cells outside the body, which suggests that it may also inhibit the growth of cells on its own.

Selenium

FACTS

It wasn't until the 1950s that researchers recognized that this mineral played a vital role in the human body. In recent years, selenium has become a superstar among minerals because of its reputed ability to prevent cancer and heart disease.

Selenium is an antioxidant. It works with glutathione peroxidase to prevent damage by free radicals. Selenium is also involved in the metabolism of prostaglandins, hormonelike substances used by the body in many different ways.

In the body, selenium detoxifies metals, such as arsenic and mercury, that would otherwise be lethal.

Selenium is synergistic with vitamin E, which means that the two combined increase the potency of each other.

Good food sources of selenium include garlic, onions, tuna, herring, broccoli, wheat germ, whole grains, sesame seeds, red grapes, egg yolks, and mushrooms. The selenium content in food varies from region to region due to differing levels of selenium in the soil.

THE RIGHT AMOUNT

The recommended daily allowance is 50 to 100 micrograms. I recommend 200 micrograms daily. Some cancer researchers feel that 300 micrograms per day is needed. Selenium can be toxic in high doses; therefore, do not exceed 300 micrograms daily. (Studies have shown that toxicity may occur at levels of 2400 micrograms daily for a prolonged period of time. However, I suggest that we err on the side of caution until we know precisely what levels are safe.)

POSSIBLE BENEFITS

Cancer Fighter • Population studies show that the rate of cancer deaths can be directly correlated to the selenium intake in food: people who eat the least amount of selenium have the highest rates of cancer. For example, in Japan where the daily selenium intake is 500 micrograms, the cancer rate is more than five times lower than it is in countries where the selenium intake is half that amount. Researchers have also found higher blood levels of selenium in healthy people as opposed to cancer patients.

Many animal studies confirm that selenium can prevent cancerous growths. Some studies show that selenium actually protects cell membranes from attack by free radicals that may explain its ability to ward off cancer.

Cardiovascular Health • Selenium may also protect lipids from oxidation, a process that may contribute to the formation of atherosclerotic lesions in the coronary arteries. Selenium may also help to prevent blood clots which can cause a stroke. Studies have linked a low selenium intake to a higher rate of both heart attack and stroke. In Colorado Springs, Colorado, which can boast the highest selenium soil content in the United States, the death rate due to heart disease is 67 percent below the national average.

Anti-inflammatory • Selenium appears to have some anti-inflammatory properties. In fact, selenium in combination with vitamin E has been used to treat arthritis in animal studies. Some people swear that selenium can help reduce the pain and stiffness of arthritis.

Male Potency • Men need this mineral! Selenium is necessary for sperm production. Almost half of a male's supply of selenium is concentrated in the testicles and portions of the seminal ducts adjacent to the prostate gland. Selenium is reputed to increase the male sex drive.

Sesame

FACTS

No reputable Asian chef would be caught without his or her bottle of sesame oil, a commonly used seasoning in the Orient. Asians may use sesame oil because of its delicate, nutty flavor. Westerners, however, may turn to sesame oil as a painless way to help prevent cancer and heart disease.

THE RIGHT AMOUNT

Sprinkle a few drops of sesame oil in stir-fry dishes.

POSSIBLE BENEFITS

Cancer Fighter • Sesame seeds and oil are an excellent source of phytic acid, an antioxidant that may prevent the kind of cellular damage that can lead to cancer. In addition, Japanese studies have shown that sesame oil may protect against colon cancer. In animal studies, sesame oil added to the diet of rats reduced the amount of bile acids in the feces. Bile acids are believed to produce cancerous changes in cells of the intestinal wall, which could cause colon cancer.

Heart Disease • Sesamin, a lignin from sesame oil, significantly reduced the amount of serum and liver cholesterol in rats fed a normal diet. Researchers speculate that sesamin may help keep cholesterol levels under control in humans.

Solanaceous Foods

FACTS

Mediterranean countries, such as Crete and Greece, have a much lower rate of heart disease and cancer than Western countries. Perhaps these countries can attribute their good health to their high intake of solanaceous foods. The solanaceous family, which includes tomatoes, eggplant, and peppers, is being investigated by the National Cancer Institute for its potential cancer-preventive properties. These foods are a mainstay of Mediterranean cuisine and are found in abundance in nearly every meal. Solanaceous foods are also an excellent source of vitamins, minerals, and fiber.

THE RIGHT AMOUNT

I recommend eating at least one serving of solanceous food daily. You can't get these critical phytochemicals in a vitamin pill; you must eat the whole food!

Caution: Some people with arthritis may find that peppers and tomatoes may aggravate their condition.

POSSIBLE BENEFITS

Cancer Fighter   •   Out of the fourteen possible phytochemicals known or believed to possess anticancer activity, the solanaceous family has seven of these important compounds including flavonoids, glucarates, carotenoids, courmarins, monoterpenes, triterpenes, and phenolic acids. Researchers believe that each of these compounds may intercede at various stages of cancer development. Some compounds may block a carcinogen that can initiate cancer, that is, a substance that alters a healthy cell, making it susceptible to cancerous growth. Others may block a cancer promoter, the substance that stimulates the altered cell to grow.

Soybeans

FACTS

For a book full of information about these wonderful legumes, see *Earl Mindell's Soy Miracle*. The National Cancer Institute is giving top priority to investigating the potential cancer-fighting properties of soybeans, and several studies have shown that soy may protect against heart disease. Anyone who wants to live longer should be eating this food.

The Japanese, who live longer than any other nationality on earth, eat lots of soy. In fact, by the turn of the century, 20 percent of all Japanese will be sixty-five or over as compared with about 13 percent of people in the United States. Some researchers believe that Japanese longevity may be due to the fact that the typical Japanese diet is rich in soy foods, products derived from soybeans. Tofu, a bean curd made from dried soybeans, and miso, a soup made from soy paste, are staples in the Japanese diet.

Ironically, the United States—not Japan—is the world's leading producer of soy. Although soy is not as popular in the United States as it is in Japan, soy-based foods are popping up in natural food stores and supermarkets across the country. Rich in protein, soy is an extremely versatile food that can be used in many different ways. Soy milk is used in formula for infants who are allergic to cow's milk. Rehydrated textured vegetable protein, a soy product sold in natural food stores, can be used as a substitute for ground beef in dishes such as chili or tacos. Soy flour can be used to make everything from muffins to pancakes. Tofu, which is flavorless and odorless, assumes the flavor of other foods and spices and can be made into everything from a frozen dessert resembling ice cream to a mock egg salad.

THE RIGHT AMOUNT

I recommend eating at least one soy product daily, and substituting soy milk for cow's milk. I make a soy milk shake for breakfast every morning.

POSSIBLE BENEFITS

Heart Disease • Recent studies show that adding soy to your diet may be one of the most effective ways to lower cholesterol. A group headed by researcher Susan M. Potter at the University of Illinois at Urbana-Champaign, tested the effects of soy protein consumption on twenty-six men with moderately high cholesterol. The men replaced 50 percent of their normal daily protein consumption with 50 grams of soy protein. The protein was baked into foods such as muffins, cookies, and breads. At the end of 4 weeks, each man had an average reduction in total cholesterol of 12 percent, thus reducing their risk of heart disease by 25 percent.

Although soy is not typically used as a cholesterol-lowering treatment in the United States, according to Dr. Potter, it is the primary cholesterol reduction treatment in Italy. Based on the study at the University of Illinois, it appears as if soy protein may be as effective a treatment as some of the medications that are prescribed for hypercholesterolemia, which have many dangerous and unpleasant side effects. If you have high cholesterol, you may want to talk to your doctor about trying a soy regime before taking medication.

Cancer Fighter • There are several compounds in soy that may help to prevent cancer. Soy contains phytochemicals called *lignans* and *isoflavonoids,* two compounds that are converted in the intestine into an estrogenlike substance called *ekuol.* Ekuol competes with a more potent form of estrogen, estradiol, for space on estrogen receptors on some cells. If the estradiol has no place to bind, it becomes deactivated. Many researchers believe that estradiol promotes the growth of tumors, especially in the breast. (Japanese women, who typically eat lots of soy, have a much lower rate of breast cancer than American women. In Japan, 6 out of 100,000 women will develop breast cancer in their lifetime versus 24 out of 100,000 in the United States.)

Soy may have a similar effect on the hormonal balance in men: American men are four times more likely to develop cancer of the prostate than Japanese men. Prostate cancer is believed to be caused by high levels of a potent form of testosterone, which may be deactivated by lignans and isoflavonoids. There may be other factors contributing to the disparity in cancer rates—Japanese men eat a diet that is much lower in fat and red meat—however, the phytochemicals in soy may also offer some protection.

Genistein is another compound in soy that is believed to be a potent cancer fighter. Genistein blocks angiogenesis, the process in which new blood vessels grow, thus literally "starving" malignant tumors from the nutrients needed to help them grow.

Menopause • In Japan, hot flashes and other unpleasant symptoms of menopause due to lower estrogen levels are a rarity. In fact, few Japanese women take estrogen replacement therapy, a common treatment for menopause in the United States. Soy researcher Herman Aldercreutz of the University of Helsinki suggested in a letter to *The New England Journal of Medicine* that the hormonelike properties of the phytochemicals in soy may be one reason why Japanese women have an easier time with menopause than American women.

Sulforaphane

FACTS

Sulforaphane is a *phytochemical,* a biologically active compound found in many cruciferous vegetables (e.g., broccoli, brussels sprouts, kale, and cauliflower) and also in carrots and green onions. According to researchers at Johns Hopkins School of Medicine, sulforaphane may be the most powerful natural anti-cancer compound discovered to date.

THE RIGHT AMOUNT

There is no recommended daily allowance for sulforaphane. I recommend two servings (2 cups) of sulforaphane-rich foods daily.

POSSIBLE BENEFITS

Cancer Fighter • Vegetables contain chemicals that promote the formation of different enzymes in humans. Some of these enzymes (phase I) are "bad guys": they actually convert benign substances into oxidants, which can damage a cell's DNA, thus promoting the risk of cancer. In response to the oxidant threat, cells can also make phase II enzymes, the so-called good guys who protect the cells' vulnerable genetic material from the bad guys. Many foods, such as hamburger, cause cells to create both good and bad enzymes. However, researchers at Johns Hopkins discovered that sulforaphane promotes the production of only phase II good enzymes, thus helping the body to ward off potential carcinogens. Although there may be other foods that also trigger the production of only phase II enzymes, the researchers suspect that sulforaphane may create even higher levels of good enzymes than these other foods.

In animal studies, sulforaphane has been shown to protect against cancer. In one study, scientists pretreated twenty-nine rats with a synthetic version of sulforaphane and then injected them with a carcinogen known to induce mammary tumors. The scientists then injected twenty-five other rats with the carcinogen without pretreating them with the sulforaphane. More than two-thirds of the group that did not receive the sulforaphane treatment eventually developed mammary cancers as opposed to only 35 percent of the group that received a low dose of sulforaphane. Out of the rats that received a high dose of sulforaphane, only 26 percent went on to develop cancer. More studies are needed to determine if sulforaphane will have the same effect on women.

Thiamine (Vitamin B_1)

FACTS

Thiamine, known as vitamin B_1, breaks down and converts carbohydrates into glucose, which provides energy for the body. Thiamine is necessary for the normal functioning of the nervous system, heart, and other muscles.

Gross thiamine deficiency will lead to beriberi, a life-threatening disease that commonly used to afflict sailors. Today, beriberi is rare; however, mild thiamine deficiency is common among older people.

Mild thiamine deficiency can lead to lack of energy, moodiness, numbness in the legs, mild depression, loss of appetite, and a general apathy among other symptoms.

Good food sources of thiamine include brewer's yeast, rice husks, unrefined cereal grains, sunflower seeds, pecans, lean pork, green peas, organic meats, most vegetables, and milk. However, thiamine is easily destroyed by exposure to light and heat.

THE RIGHT AMOUNT

The recommended daily allowance for thiamine for adults is 1.0 to 1.5 milligrams. Thiamine can be destroyed by alcohol; alcoholics and heavy drinkers are at risk of thiamine deficiency. Thiamine is usually included in B-complex supplements and multivitamins.

If you use antacids or aspirin on a regular basis, you may need extra thiamine.

Thiamine has no known toxic effects.

POSSIBLE BENEFITS

Heart Disease • Thiamine is essential for the normal function of the heart. Serious thiamine deficiencies may lead to potentially fatal heart arrhythmias and heart failure. Given the fact that heart disease is the number one killer in the United States and studies show that thiamine deficiency is not uncommon among the elderly, it's critical for older adults to maintain normal thiamine levels.

Antistress • In times of physical or emotional stress, your intake of B vitamins, including thiamine, should be increased. In my experience, many people find that thiamine along with other B vitamins can help alleviate symptoms of stress such as mild depression.

Tocopherol (Vitamin E)

FACTS

A physician friend who is highly skeptical about all forms of vitamin supplements recently confessed that she is beginning to have second thoughts about vitamin E. "I've noticed that among my older patients, those who take vitamin E are the most together, healthiest people in my practice," she said. "It finally dawned on me that there must be something to this vitamin E."

A lot of people, many of them M.D.s, have reached the same conclusion. Sales of vitamin E have soared, and it is now enjoying superstar status among its fellow micronutrients. However, vitamin E is no overnight success; it took more than 70 years for the medical community to begin to take it seriously.

Vitamin E was first discovered in 1922 when researchers noticed, quite by accident, that rats could not breed without it. They dubbed this substance *tocopherol,* from the Greek "to bring forth in childbirth." They are actually eight different types of tocopherol, of which alpha-tocopherol is the most effective.

Vitamin E is a fat-soluble vitamin, which means that unlike water-soluble vitamins, it is not excreted in the urine, but stored in the liver.

Vitamin E is potent antioxidant; it has been dubbed the body's first line of defense against lipid peroxidation—that means it protects polyunsaturated fatty acids in the cell membrane from free radical attack.

Vitamin E is found in vegetable oils, whole grains, sweet potatoes, wheat germ, brown rice, nuts, and other foods.

Vitamin E is synergistic with selenium (another Hot 100 antioxidant), which means that the two combined greatly enhance each other's potency.

THE RIGHT AMOUNT

The recommended daily allowance for vitamin E is 8 to 10 international units; however supplements usually come in 100-international-unit strength. I recommend at least 400–800 international units of vitamin E daily. (With this vitamin, 1 international unit is equivalent to 1 milligram.)

Caution: Do not take vitamin E if you are taking a blood thinner such as aspirin or have vitamin K deficiency. If you've had a bleeding problem in the past, talk to your physician before taking vitamin E.

POSSIBLE BENEFITS

Heart Disease • In the 1970s, two Canadian physicians, Drs. Wilfred and Evan Shute, promoted vitamin E as a weapon against heart disease in their best-selling book, *Vitamin E for Ailing and Healthy Hearts*. Most cardiologists ridiculed the notion that a mere vitamin could be a powerful heart medicine. They're no longer laughing. Several recent studies have shown that a link between daily vitamin E consumption and a lowered risk of heart disease in both men and women. In May 1993, *The New England Journal of Medicine* reported the results of an 8-year study involving more than 87,000 registered female nurses and a related study involving close to 40,000 male health professionals. In both studies, participants who consumed vitamin E supplements (of at least 100 international units or more) for a minimum of 2 years had a 40 percent lower risk of heart disease than those who derived vitamin E through diet alone. At first, researchers suspected that people taking vitamin E may be more health conscious and therefore have healthier habits, which could also account for the reduction in heart disease. However, even after factoring in lifestyle, the vitamin E supplement appeared to be the primary difference between the group who developed heart disease and the group who remained disease free.

In another study sponsored by the American Heart Association, researchers found that long-term supplementation with high doses of vitamin E (160 milligrams) decreased the susceptibility of low-density lipoproteins, or "bad" cholesterol, to oxidation by 30 to 50 percent. (When low-density lipoproteins oxidize, they may contribute to the formation of atherosclerotic lesions in arteries supplying blood to the heart and other vital organs. A heart attack occurs when blood supply is cut off from the heart.)

Vitamin E is also a natural blood thinner and may prevent the formation of blood clots. If a clot enters the bloodstream and lodges in an artery feeding the brain, it could result in a stroke; if the clot lodges into a coronary artery, it could result in a heart attack.

Many cardiac surgeons give coronary bypass patients high doses of vitamin E prior to surgery. A recent study of coronary bypass patients performed at the Mayo Clinic in Rochester, Minnesota, found that patients given 2000 international units of vitamin E prior to surgery had much lower blood levels of free radicals after surgery than patients who had not been given the supplemental E. They also found that patients who had been given additional vitamin E had normal blood levels of E following surgery, whereas the unsupplemented patients had lower than normal levels.

Cancer Fighter • There is growing evidence that vitamin E may protect against various forms of cancer. A study sponsored by the National Cancer Institute suggests that people who take a vitamin E supplement for a minimum of six months cut their risk of developing oral cancers in half. Factors known to increase the risk of oral cancers, such as alcohol consumption, smoking, and dietary habits, made no difference in the outcome. These findings are consistent with animal studies that showed that vitamin E reduced the effects of carcinogens on cheek cells in hamsters.

Another study performed at the Biodynamics Institute at Louisiana State University showed that vitamin E may protect humans against the harmful effects of chronic exposure to ozone in smog. The study suggests that vitamin E's potent antioxidant activity may guard against the biological damage inflicted by ozone on lung tissue.

Vitamin E may also help to prevent stomach cancer and other cancers of the gastrointestinal tract by inhibiting the conversion of nitrates, which are found in food, to nitrosamines in the stomach. Nitrosamines are potentially carcinogenic.

Diabetes • In a recent Italian study, daily vitamin E supplements (900 milligrams for 4 months) helped people with type II diabetes better use insulin. Type II diabetes—also known as adult- or late-onset diabetes—accounts for 90 percent of all cases of diabetes and occurs during middle age and beyond. People with this form of diabetes can develop dangerously high levels of glucose in the blood. Based on this study, vitamin E appeared to help maintain normal blood glucose levels. (If you have diabetes, check with your physician before using vitamin E or any other medication.)

Immunity • Studies have shown that older people with low blood serum levels of vitamin E are more vulnerable to developing infections. A recent study in *The American Journal of Clinical Nutrition* showed that short-term supplementation with high doses of vitamin E can enhance immune responsiveness in healthy individuals over sixty. In the study, thirty-two healthy older adults who were not taking any vitamin supplements or prescription medication were either given 800 milligrams of vitamin E daily for 3 days or a placebo. Based on blood and skin tests, those taking the vitamin E showed a dramatic boost in immune function. Those taking the placebo did not show any change. Considering the fact that immune function declines as we age, this is a particularly important finding.

Brain • Researchers at the Neurological Institute at Columbia University College of Physicians and Surgeons in New York gave patients with tardive dyskinesia (a neurological disorder that can result from long-term use of antipsychotic medications) vitamin E supplements along with antipsychotic medications. The group taking the vitamin E showed improvement in tremors and a reduction in anxiety and depression. Researchers are considering using antioxidant vitamins including E on patients with Parkinson's disease, another neurologic disorder that often affects the elderly.

Skin • For decades, vitamin E fans have claimed that if used directly on the skin, vitamin E oil can help prevent the signs of aging. A recent study suggests that vitamin E may reduce the severity of wrinkles. In the study, twenty middle-aged women were given a 5 percent strength cream of vitamin E to put on their skin daily. At the end of 4 weeks, the women showed a 50 percent reduction in the length and depth of crow's feet; although the wrinkles were still there, they looked better. However, many cosmetic creams that tout vitamin E as an ingredient actually contain very little E. Use only creams that list vitamin E or tocopherol near the top of the ingredient list, which means that it is a primary ingredient. Do not use the oil from the vitamin E capsule directly on the skin; it can cause irritation in many people.

Protects Against Muscle Damage • Although vigorous exercise is good for your heart, it may also promote muscle damage due to oxidation. (Remember, as you exercise, your body's demand for oxygen increases—the more oxygen, the greater the risk of oxidation.) However, according to a study at the Human Nutrition Research Center on Aging at Tufts University, a daily vitamin E supplement may help protect against free radical damage caused by working out.

Eyes • Researchers suspect that cataracts, which cloud the eye lens, may be caused by oxidative damage to the lens covering of the eye and that vitamin E may help protect the eye from this kind of damage. A recent study suggests that they may be right. Finnish researchers discovered that people with low blood serum levels of vitamin E (and also beta-carotene, another member of the Hot 100) were twice as likely to develop cataracts as those with higher levels.

Arthritis • Studies suggest that vitamin E supplements may relieve some of the symptoms of osteoarthritis. Arthritis has been associated with elevated levels of free radicals.

Anecdotal Evidence • Many people swear that vitamin E helps to prevent their hair from turning gray. Recently, an Ohio physician even wrote a letter to the *New York Times* describing how he and his patients keep their hair from turning gray by taking vitamin E. Although there's no evidence to prove that vitamin E helps to keep the gray away, I've heard it from enough people to make me wonder whether there's any truth to it.

Tretinoin

FACTS

Marketed under the name Retin-A, tretinoin, a form of topical vitamin A, was approved by the Food and Drug Administration over 20 years ago as a treatment for severe acne. Dermatologists observed that this cream not only helped rid their patients of acne, but it also appeared to help erase fine lines and wrinkles. By the late 1980s, tretinoin was being touted as a miracle cream, and it quickly became one of the most frequently prescribed topical medications. In recent years, tretinoin has been eclipsed by the growing popularity of alpha-hydroxy acids and other hot, new "cosmetceuticals." Tretinoin has its shortcomings: its effectiveness peaks after about 24 months of use. In addition, if you stop using it, the changes begin to fade. Despite these problems, tretinoin is still one of the most effective anti-aging skin products on the market.

THE RIGHT AMOUNT

Apply cream as directed by your physician.

Caution: Most users experience skin peeling or irritation at least initially. Tretinoin must be used in conjunction with a sunscreen because it makes the skin more prone to sun damage. High doses of oral vitamin A have been associated with birth defects. Although there is no evidence that topical vitamin A can cause similar problems, women who are pregnant or trying to conceive should not use tretinoin.

POSSIBLE BENEFITS

Skin Rejuvenator • As we age, skin tends to thin out and become dryer. Wrinkles develop when collagen and elastin, proteins in the skin that provide elasticity, begin to break down. Studies have shown that tretinoin can increase skin thickness, improve circulation, and increase collagen. (Collagen is the "glue" that holds cells together.) Tretinoin appears to help plump out the skin, erasing fine lines and wrinkles. After about 6 weeks of use, many people find that their skin looks pinker and fresher. (However, tretinoin is ineffective against deep wrinkles.)

Turmeric

FACTS

Turmeric is an herb that adds flavor and color to many foods, including curry powder and sauces. In the West, turmeric has been used primarily as a spice. In Asia, however, this herb has a rich medicinal history. Westerners are just beginning to discover this herb's potential as a longevity booster.

Turmeric is a "heart healthy" herb that may help prevent heart disease. It is also a natural anti-inflammatory.

THE RIGHT AMOUNT

Turmeric is available in capsule and tablet form. Take 1 to 3 capsules or tablets daily.

POSSIBLE BENEFITS

Heart Disease   •   Studies show that turmeric can lower blood cholesterol levels. Turmeric stimulates the production of bile by the liver. Cholesterol is a component of bile, thus, when the liver produces bile, it utilizes excess cholesterol.

Turmeric also prevents the formation of dangerous blood clots that can lead to heart attack or stroke. In fact, as Daniel Mowrey noted in his book, *Next Generation Herbal Medicine*, people who live in countries where curry is frequently eaten have a much lower level of thrombosis (blood clots) than people who live in Western countries.

Arthritis   •   Traditional healers have used turmeric to reduce the inflammation and pain associated with arthritis. Based on anecdotal evidence, I believe that some people may find that turmeric may indeed help control arthritis.

Umbelliferous Vegetables

FACTS

In an article that appeared in *Food Technology*, Alegria Caragay, Ph.D., an advisor to the Designer Food Program for the National Cancer Institute (NCI), wrote, "Within the last decade, as research into the relationship between diet and cancer has proliferated, so, too, has the body of data from both epidemiological and animal studies that indicates vegetables, grains, and fruits may contain certain cancer-preventing substances." In the article, Dr. Caragay noted that umbelliferous vegetables were at the top of the NCI's list of foods with potentially important anticancer properties. In fact, the NCI is pouring millions of dollars into researching these foods.

Umbelliferous vegetables include carrots, celery, and parsnips.

THE RIGHT AMOUNT

Umbelliferous vegetables contain six important phytochemicals that may help prevent cancer and heart disease. You can't get these compounds in a pill, you must eat the whole food. People who want to live longer and live healthier should make sure that umbelliferous vegetables are included in their diets.

POSSIBLE BENEFITS

Cancer Fighter • Umbelliferous vegetables contain compounds that can thwart the initiation and spread of cancer such as the following:

> *Flavonoids.* These compounds help protect cell membranes against oxidation and may deactivate potent hormones that can trigger the growth of tumors.
> *Carotenoids.* These compounds help protect cells against oxidative damage that can damage DNA.
> *Coumarins.* These compounds may block the action of car-

cinogens before they can damage healthy cells, which can cause these cells to mutate.

Phenolic acids. These compounds may block the action of hormonelike compounds called *prostagladins,* which can promote the growth of tumors.

Heart Disease • Umbelliferous vegetables are rich in antioxidants—carotenoids such as beta-carotene, flavonoids, and phenolic acids. Studies have shown that people who take antioxidants daily have lower rates of heart disease than those who do not. Researchers believe that antioxidants may prevent the oxidation of low-density lipoproteins, or "bad" cholesterol, which may promote atherosclerosis, or hardening of the arteries.

Vitex

FACTS

Vitex, an herb that dates back to ancient times, is being rediscovered by a generation of modern women who are seeking a natural approach to menopause. Also called *chaste tree* or *chasteberry,* vitex was used by the early Greeks who believed that it could dampen sexual desire. According to *The New Age Herbalist,* in Italy the flowers of this plant are still strewn in the path of novices when they first enter the monastery or convent, presumably because of vitex's reputation as an anti-aphrodisiac. Folklore aside, there is no evidence that vitex has any effect whatsoever on libido; however, this herb does appear to have a positive effect on the female reproductive system and is used to treat a wide variety of "female complaints."

THE RIGHT AMOUNT

Vitex is available in capsule form at natural food stores. Take 1 capsule up to three times daily. Vitex is also included in many herbal formulas for women.

POSSIBLE BENEFITS

Menopause • Herbalists have traditionally used vitex to treat symptoms associated with menstrual problems such as premenstrual syndrome. Recent studies show that vitex is a *hormone regulator*. It increases production of luteinizing hormone, inhibits production of follicle-stimulating hormone, and may stimulate the production of progesterone. The overall effect of vitex is to prevent the kind of hormonal fluctuations that can cause some very annoying symptoms during menopause such as hot flashes and irritability.

Water

FACTS

Most of us take water for granted, and yet, we couldn't live without it for more than a few days. Water is involved in nearly every bodily process. In fact, water is the most abundant fluid in the human body, accounting for one-half to two-thirds of total body weight.

Nutrients and hormones circulate throughout the body via water. Water also improves kidney function, which tends to decline with age. In addition, water cushions or lubricates joints and prevents friction between bones and ligaments.

Water is also an excellent source of minerals such as calcium, magnesium, and selenium. The rate of cardiovascular disease is higher in areas with "soft water," that is, where the water contains low levels of minerals such as magnesium and calcium.

As we age, our sensation of thirst becomes somewhat blunted, which increases the risk of not drinking enough fluids.

Good sources of water include drinking water, juices, milk, fruits, and vegetables. Watermelon, lettuce, cucumbers, and celery are especially good sources.

THE RIGHT AMOUNT

I advise 6 to 8 glasses of water daily. Be sure to drink water even if you're not thirsty.

Caution: Unfortunately, not all water is pure and healthy. In some cases, water may be tainted with lead from old pipes. In other areas, high levels of chlorine and other potential toxins may make water unsafe. If you live in an area where the water is suspect, I recommend installing a home filtering system or using bottled water for drinking.

If you use a home filtering system, remember that it must be properly maintained and checked periodically. Activated carbon filters must be changed every few months or they can develop harmful contaminants. If you have a reverse osmosis system (which removes chemicals but not necessarily all inorganic contaminants), be sure to test it periodically because the filter can become tainted with bacteria. In addition, distillers, which are excellent for removing inorganic contaminants (but not quite as good for organic contaminants), must be descaled regularly.

Depending on processing techniques, not all bottled water is safe either. To ensure purity, try to use only water that has undergone the process of reverse osmosis, distillation, or a combination of reverse osmosis and deionization. Stick to well-known or national brands.

POSSIBLE BENEFITS

Prevents Constipation   •   Older Americans spend millions of dollars a year on laxatives. Drinking 6 to 8 glasses of water per day will help to increase intestinal motility and prevent constipation.

Weight Control   •   Instead of reaching for something to eat, try drinking a glass of water. If you're dieting, drink a glass or two of water before meals to curb your appetite. Water fills you up without filling you out.

Skin • As we age, sweat and oil glands, which moisturize skin, begin to slow down. The top layer of skin begins to thin, which makes it more difficult for skin to retain its natural moisture, resulting in drier, older-looking skin. In addition, if you don't replace fluid lost to urination and sweat, your body will pull fluid from other body cells, including skin cells. Drinking water can help your skin retain some of its youthful freshness.

PERSONAL ADVICE

If you're running a fever, you need to be sure to drink enough water. In addition, caffeine is a natural diuretic that can increase water loss. If you drink a lot of coffee, tea, or colas with caffeine, be sure to increase your water intake.

If you want to test your tap water for lead, the Environmental Protection Agency's Drinking Water Hot Line (800-426-4791) will refer you to a certified lab in your area. Most labs will send a kit in the mail. (Prices range from fifteen to thirty dollars.)

Wheat Bran

FACTS

All bran is not the same. Researchers are discovering that different kinds of bran perform different functions in the body. Some types of bran are particularly good at lowering cholesterol, others promote bowel regularity. Because of its unique properties, wheat bran may protect against two common forms of cancer: breast cancer and colon cancer.

Good sources of wheat bran include whole wheat bread and cereals. Wheat bran can also be added to hot cereal or baked foods or mixed in yogurt.

THE RIGHT AMOUNT

I recommend one or two servings of a food rich in wheat bran daily.

POSSIBLE BENEFITS

Breast Cancer • Higher levels of circulating estrogen is believed to be a risk factor for developing breast cancer. Recently, researchers at the American Health Foundation studied the effect of three different types of bran (oat, corn, and wheat) on the estrogen levels of sixty-two premenopausal women. Participants were randomly selected to receive either a wheat, oat, or corn bran supplement in the form of food. For each woman, the average daily fiber intake was increased from about 15 to 30 percent. After 2 months, the women taking the corn or oat bran showed no change in estrogen levels. The women eating the diet rich in wheat bran, however, showed significant reductions in serum estrone, a potent form of estrogen that may promote the growth of estrogen-sensitive tumors.

Colon Cancer • Colon cancer is one of the leading causes of death in the United States annually, accounting for more than sixty thousand fatalities. Although some forms of colon cancer may be genetic, most appear to be due to diet and environmental factors. A recent study at New York Hospital/Cornell Medical Center suggests that wheat bran may play an important in preventing this disease. In the study, fifty-eight people with precancerous polyps were divided into two groups. One group was put on a high-fiber diet rich in wheat bran cereal. The other group was given a low-fiber cereal. Most of the people eating the wheat bran experienced a reduction in the size and number of their polyps. There was no change seen in those on the low-fiber diet.

White Willow

FACTS

For thousands of years, the bark of this tree has been used to treat pain and fever. White willow bark contains salicin, a compound that provided chemists with the model for acetylsalicyclic acid—better known as aspirin. White willow is similar to aspirin in activity but is weaker. Unlike aspirin, which can cause stomach irritation, white willow also contains tannins, which aid in digestion.

THE RIGHT AMOUNT

White willow is available as capsules at natural food stores. Take 1 or 2 capsules every 3 to 4 hours as needed.

POSSIBLE BENEFITS

Arthritis • About 20 million Americans suffer from arthritis, which literally means inflammation of a joint. Arthritis is a common ailment, especially among older women. In fact, some 10 million women suffer from this problem. There are many different forms of arthritis, and symptoms may vary. However, typical symptoms include aches and pains in joints and connective tissue throughout the body. Aspirin and other anti-inflammatory medications are prescribed as the first line of defense against this disease. As good as these drugs may be, many have some very unpleasant and potentially dangerous side effects including gastrointestinal distress and bleeding. For many people, white willow bark works as well as aspirin in controlling pain but without the side effects.

PERSONAL ADVICE

Herbal medications may take longer to work than stronger drugs. Use this herb for 2 weeks to see if it helps control your symptoms.

Wild Yam

FACTS

Wild yam, often touted as the hot anti-aging herb of the future, has an interesting past. For generations, southern blacks have used the root of this plant to treat rheumatoid arthritis and colic. Female herbalists have routinely prescribed it for menstrual disorders including premenstrual syndrome and threatened miscarriage. In 1943, wild yam attracted the attention of mainstream medicine when a scientist extracted the female hormone progesterone from this plant. In fact, until 1970, this plant was the sole source of progesterone used in birth control pills. Today, this herb is primarily used to treat two conditions associated with aging: menopause and arthritis.

THE RIGHT AMOUNT

Wild yam is available in capsule form at natural food stores. Take 1 capsule up to three times daily; I do.

POSSIBLE BENEFITS

Rheumatoid Arthritis   •   Animal studies have confirmed that the steroidal saponins in wild yam have an anti-inflammatory effect and, therefore, may be useful in treating the pain and stiffness associated with a flare-up of rheumatoid arthritis.

Menopause   •   Wild yam is believed to regulate hormonal fluctuations that can cause unpleasant menopausal symptoms such as hot flashes, fatigue, and vaginal dryness. This herb is often included in herbal formulas designed to relieve menopausal symptoms.

Yohimbe Bark

FACTS

Since ancient times, different herbs and potions have been touted as aphrodisiacs. Few of these so-called aphrodisiacs have withstood serious scientific scrutiny with the exception of yohimbe. A compound extracted from the bark of the African yohimbe tree is a proven aphrodisiac that works well for many men. In fact, it is even prescribed by physicians under the generic name yohimbine or yohimbine hydrochloride to treat cases of male impotency.

THE RIGHT AMOUNT

Yohimbine is sold by prescription only and should only be used under the supervision of a physician. If you are a man suffering from impotency, talk to your physician about this drug.

A weaker form of this drug is sold under the name yohimbe bark at many natural food stores and herb stores. Yohimbe bark is available without prescription, but it is not as effective as yohimbine. Yohimbe bark is often included in male potency formulas with other aphrodisiacs. Take 1 to 3 capsules daily.

Caution: High doses of yohimbe can cause serious side effects in some cases. Yohimbe can lower blood pressure and should not be used by people with hypotension. In addition, yohimbe should not be used by people with medical problems unless it is under the supervision of a physician.

POSSIBLE BENEFITS

Impotency • Impotency is a widespread problem for men over forty. In a recent study that appeared in *The Journal of Urology* of thirteen hundred men between the ages of forty and seventy, at least half of the men questioned claimed to have had trouble keeping an erection within the past six months. Animal and human studies have shown that in many cases, impotency caused by either psychological or physical problems can be successfully treated with prescription strength yohimbine. For example, in one Canadian study, forty-eight men were either given a placebo or yohimbine over a 10-week period. Of those taking the yohimbine, 46 percent reported a positive response.

Zinc

FACTS

In the not too distant future, a whole population of aging baby boomers may view this common mineral with new respect. In the body, zinc performs many vital roles involving cell division, growth, and repair—all of which are functions that tend to slow down with age. Men in particular may become interested in zinc. There is a heavy concentration of zinc in the male prostate gland. Many people—myself included—suspect that zinc may help to prevent prostate problems in older men. Last but not least, recent studies suggest that zinc may be an immune booster and may even help to preserve vision in the elderly.

Marginal zinc deficiency is widespread in the United States among people of all ages, but especially among older adults. On average, women consume 70 percent of the recommended daily allowance (RDA) for zinc; men consume 90 percent.

Good sources of zinc include oysters, pork, liver, eggs, brewers yeast, milk, beans, wheat germ, and pumpkin seeds.

THE RIGHT AMOUNT

The RDA for women is 12 milligrams; the RDA for men is 15 milligrams. Zinc is available in multivitamin and multimineral preparations. Zinc gluconate and zinc picolinate appear to be the most easily tolerated. Supplements range from 15 to 60 milligrams daily. I do not recommend exceeding 50 milligrams daily. Very high doses of zinc (over 150 milligrams) may actually depress the immune system. Excess zinc may also impair copper absorption.

POSSIBLE BENEFITS

Immune Enhancer • Several studies have been done on the role of zinc deficiency in the immune function of older people. One recent study showed that zinc supplements (220 milligrams twice daily for 1 month) increased the level of T cells in people over seventy. (T cells help fight infection.)

Cold Fighter • Move over vitamin C—zinc may be a more potent cold fighter. In a study, seventy-three Dartmouth College students with colds were given zinc lozenges (zinc–gluconate–glycine) at the earliest stages of the illness. The lozenges reduced the duration of colds by more than 40 percent (from an average of 9 days to 5 days) and also greatly reduced the severity of cold symptoms. The students sucked on 2 lozenges every 2 hours, up to 8 per day. (Zinc lozenges should not be taken on an empty stomach because they can cause nausea.)

Vision • Macular degeneration, which causes a blur or blind spot in the field of vision, is a common malady of aging, which, in some cases, can be treated surgically. In one small study performed at Louisiana State University Medical Center, zinc supplements appeared to help control vision loss due to macular degeneration. In the study, 151 patients were given either 100-milligram tablets of zinc twice daily or a placebo. Those who were given the zinc showed in the words of the researchers "significantly less visual loss" than the placebo group. The National Eye Institute in Bethesda is embarking on a 6-year study to determine the role nutrition and supplements such as zinc may play in the progression of eye diseases such as macular degeneration and cataracts. Perhaps by the twenty-first century, we'll have some definitive answers.

Prostate • For years, I've been recommending zinc supplements to men with prostate problems. There are heavy concentrations of zinc in the male prostate gland, which manufactures prostatic fluid, in which sperm cells are mixed to make semen.

There is a great deal of anecdotal evidence supporting zinc's role in prostate health and male infertility. However, few scientific studies have been done. In fact, recently, in the *Nutrition Action Healthletter* published by the Center for Science in the Public Interest, there was an interesting letter to the editor responding to an article in the newsletter that had stated that there was no scientific evidence linking zinc intake to prostate health. In the letter, a California man pointed out that he was one of three brothers, all in their midsixties. One brother was a regular user of zinc for 30 years, the others were not. The two brothers who did not use zinc had developed enlarged prostates and even cancer; the zinc user had not. Coincidence? Maybe. But I've heard enough of these kinds of stories to make sure that I get enough zinc daily!

Up and Coming Supplements

Here are some potentially beneficial anti-aging supplements that are the focus of several research projects. I predict that you'll be hearing a lot more about them in the near future.

DEHYDROEPIANDROSTERONE

Dehydroepiandrosterone (DHEA) is a hormone that is produced by the adrenal glands. DHEA is abundant in the young, but in middle age, the supply begins to drop. By age fifty, most people produce only one-third of the DHEA that they did in their youth. By age sixty, DHEA levels are barely detectable.

Some researchers believe that the precipitous drop in DHEA makes people more vulnerable to many of the ailments that are often associated with old age, including two of the leading killers of both men and women: cancer and heart disease.

In one long-term study of men between the ages of fifty and seventy-nine, researchers found that those with the lowest levels of DHEA had the highest rate of heart disease. Other studies of healthy men suggest that DHEA supplements can cut cholesterol, reduce body fat, increase muscle mass, and relieve depression. Animal studies have shown that DHEA supplements can thwart the growth of artificially planted tumors in elderly mice. In addition, DHEA can help improve memory, at least in laboratory mice, and may even make it easier to lose weight.

DHEA may sound like a wonder drug but like other forms of hormone therapy, it has its downside. In very high doses DHEA can cause the overproduction of sex hormones and liver enlargement. In women, DHEA can have an androgenic effect, which means it can produce some unwanted side affects such as a growth spurt in facial hair. Human studies are being conducted to determine what levels of supplemental DHEA are safe for humans and whether DHEA is truly a life extender. Dr. Arthur Schwartz, a biologist at Temple University and a leading authority on DHEA, advises people to avoid supplements until some of these questions are answered, but other proponents of DHEA feel that it is safe in low dosages.

DHEA is available only by prescription.

HUMAN GROWTH HORMONE

Human growth hormone is released by the pituitary gland until age thirty and is closely related to the stages of development. Levels of growth hormone are high in the fetus, decline during early childhood, and surge again during adolescence. (Interestingly enough, the greatest amount of growth hormone is released just before deep sleep, which could explain why adolescents seem to need so much sleep, and why children seem to grow in their sleep.) After age thirty, however, the levels of human growth hormone sharply decline and in some older persons, production seems to shut down altogether. As the level of growth hormone declines, so does body function. In fact, low levels of growth hormone have been associated with a drop in muscle mass, an increase in body fat, diminished immunologic response, a loss of appetite, and a reduction in kidney function. Some researchers have speculated that supplementing growth hormone in aging people may reverse some of these negative effects.

In 1990, Dr. Daniel Rudman of the Medical College of Wisconsin and the Milwaukee VA Medical Center assembled twenty-one healthy men, ages sixty-one to eighty-one, with one thing in common: unusually low levels of growth hormone. Twelve of the subjects received growth hormone injections over a 6-month period; nine did not. Those who received the injections had a 14 percent reduction in body fat and a 9 percent increase in muscle mass. Many of the subjects on the hormone claimed that they felt better than they had in years, and growth hormone was quickly lauded as the "fountain of youth." Once the hormone was discontinued, however, the subjects quickly returned to their original state.

So why isn't everybody popping growth hormone pills? In the United States the only medically accepted use of growth hormone is to supplement it in growing children with documented low levels. Growth hormone is available in many countries outside of the United States, and many clinics abroad are dispensing the stuff with a free hand. However, most scientists agree that more research needs to be done before growth hormone can be used by the general population. Growth hormone has some potentially hazardous side effects including cancer, arthritis, carpal tunnel syndrome, diabetes, and enlargement of the head. It can also cause swelling and headaches, even at low levels. The National Institutes of Health is funding several studies on growth hormone to determine whether it works as well as it appears, if it can be used safely, and the optimum dose.

RU-486

RU-486, or mifepristone, has gained notoriety as the so-called abortion pill. In fact, until recently, it was banned in the United States due to an extensive lobbying effort on the part of anti-abortion forces. This drug works by blocking key hormones necessary to sustain a pregnancy, including progesterone and stress hormones known as glucocorticoids. Many researchers worldwide believe that RU-486 may prove to be a real life saver.

One French study showed that RU-486 shrank tumors in 25

percent of women with advanced breast cancers. (Progesterone can stimulate the growth of tumors; therefore, any drug that can block the action of progesterone may also help prevent the growth of tumors.) More studies are being done in the United States and abroad to determine whether RU-486 could be used in the treatment or prevention of breast cancer.

Other studies suggest that RU-486 may have broader application as a general anti-aging drug. For example, in one study sponsored by the National Institute of Child Health and Human Development, RU-486 was an effective treatment for Cushing's syndrome in six out of ten children given this drug. This study caught the eye of longevity researchers primarily because the symptoms of Cushing's syndrome (which include a rapid decline in immunity, osteoporosis, and loss of muscle) closely resemble a speeded-up version of the aging process. Research is underway investigating RU-486 as a treatment for osteoporosis, high blood pressure, and adult-onset diabetes among other maladies associated with aging.

Words of Wisdom

Want to live to be one hundred and five? Follow the advice of the Delany sisters, authors of *Having Our Say: The Delany Sisters' First 100 Years.* As of this writing, Sarah L. (Sadie) Delany is one hundred and six and her sister A. Elizabeth (Bessie) Delany recently died at one hundred and four. According to the Delanys, the secret to their longevity is a combination of diet and exercise. They did yoga exercises daily and ate a clove of garlic chopped up and swallowed whole every morning with a teaspoonful of cod liver oil. In addition, the Delany sisters wrote, "We eat as many as seven different vegetables. Plus lots of fresh fruits. And we take vitamin supplements: Vitamin A, B complex, C, D, E, and minerals, too, like zinc. And Bessie takes tyrosine when she's a little blue."

Chapter 3

Living Well: A Guide to Preventing Common Ailments of Aging

Listed in this chapter are the common ailments afflicting older adults and ways that they can be prevented or treated.

Alzheimer's Disease

About 4 million Americans have Alzheimer's disease, an irreversible form of dementia that is characterized by the slow but steady destruction of key areas in the brain that control reasoning and memory. Symptoms include memory loss, the inability to speak, and difficulty in processing information. In most cases, Alzheimer's is a late-onset disease. About 10 percent of Americans over age sixty-five have Alzheimer's disease, and nearly half of those diagnosed are over eighty-five. However, about 5 percent of all Alzheimer's cases occur in people as young as forty.

Although we are quick to label any form of senility as Alzheimer's disease, in reality, there are many different types of dementia that can affect the elderly and can be caused by a wide range of factors including overmedication, stroke, poor blood flow to the brain, and even depression. In contrast, Alzheimer's is marked by specific brain abnormalities, notably, clusters of injured brain cells called *plaques,* which are believed to be responsible for the loss of memory and other behavioral abnormalities. The cause of Alzheimer's is still unknown, although it appears to be linked to certain genes. According to researchers at Duke University, people who inherit a gene that is responsible for producing a protein called Apo-E4 are four times more likely to develop Alzheimer's late in life. If they inherit the gene from both parents, the risk is doubled. (In addition, these people do not produce enough of two other proteins, Apo-E2 and Apo-E3.) However, not everyone who has these genes will get Alzheimer's, and not everyone with Alzheimer's has these genes. Other researchers believe that the culprit is actually a protein piece called *beta-amyloid peptide,* which lies at the center of the brain plaques. They suspect that this protein could be responsible for destroying brain cells.

There is no cure for Alzheimer's, and to date, drug treatments for Alzheimer's have been disappointing. However, there is strong evidence that there are simple steps that can be taken to delay the onset of Alzheimer's or to lessen the severity of the symptoms.

EARL'S RX

Use It or Lose It • Many studies have shown that people with the highest degree of education have the lowest rates of Alzheimer's disease. These results were initially chalked up to the fact that better-educated people tend to be more affluent, and more affluent people tend to take better care of themselves. However, recent research into the inner workings of the brain show that a lifetime of intellectual stimulation may have a far more profound effect. A child's brain is constantly producing new brain cells, but as we age, production of cells begins to fall off. Until recently, scientists believed that the mature brain followed a steady course of decline, but animal experiments have proved this theory wrong. Studies on rats have shown that learning new tasks can actually stimulate the production of *dendrites*, threadlike appendages at the end of brain cells called *neurons*, which helps cells communicate with each other. The growth of dendrites didn't just occur in young animals, as might be expected, but surprisingly in older animals as well. Scientists speculate that human adults who are constantly challenged by intellectual pursuits may actually be building a bigger store of dendrites than people who are not faced with intellectual challenges. Thus, it's possible that when people with a reserve of dendrites develop Alzheimer's, which slowly destroys a portion of their brains, they may not experience as severe symptoms as people with less education—and presumably fewer dendrites.

I'm not suggesting that anyone who has not attained a Ph.D. will get Alzheimer's disease. Education is not just about degrees; it's about staying interested in the world, learning new skills, and accepting new challenges at any age. Make a concerted effort to "grow your dendrites"—study a new subject, learn a new language, take up a new sport, or try your hand at painting or sculpting.

Limit Your Exposure to Aluminum • Some studies have shown high concentrations of aluminum—up to fifty times higher than normal—in some parts of the brains of Alzheimer's patients. This has led some scientists to speculate that aluminum, one of the most abundant metals on earth, may in some way be responsible for causing this disease. However, many researchers dismiss the aluminum connection, citing as evidence studies that show that people who live in areas with high levels of aluminum in their water supply do not suffer a higher rate of Alzheimer's than usual. In addition, critics of the aluminum hypothesis point out that half of all cookware used in the United States is made with aluminum, and if aluminum caused Alzheimer's, the disease would be more prevalent than it is.

Frankly, nobody knows what link, if any, exists between aluminum and Alzheimer's disease. In fact, the higher levels of aluminum found in some studies may simply be a result of the disease, not the cause. Nevertheless, I advise people to err on the side of caution. While it's impossible to avoid aluminum altogether—aluminum is present in natural sources such as fruits and vegetables and small amounts may leach from aluminum cookware into food—it is possible to avoid ingesting high doses of the metal. For example, many commonly used over-the-counter drugs such as antacids and buffered aspirin are high in aluminum. In fact, if you are a regular user of either of these products, you could be ingesting up to 5000 milligrams of aluminum daily! Many deodorants are also high in aluminum; aerosol antiperspirants may be particularly bad because anything inhaled through the nasal passages is more readily absorbed by the brain. (Fortunately, there are some excellent herbal deodorants sold at natural food stores that do not contain aluminum.) Until we know for certain that aluminum is harmless, I recommend avoiding products with a high aluminum content.

L-Carnitine • L-Carnitine (see p. 49) is a nonprotein amino acid that is found in heart and skeletal muscle. It's primary job is to carry activated fatty acids across the mitochondria—the so-called powerhouse of the cell—providing heart and skeletal cells with energy. The brain tissue of mammals is a rich source of carnitine. Some studies suggest that L-carnitine may be effective in slowing down the progression of Alzheimer's disease. Several European studies have reported that a daily supplement of L-carnitine (about 2 grams daily) can slow the mental deterioration typical of this disease. (Dietary intakes of L-Carnitine average 100 to 300 milligrams daily in the United States.) However, U.S. researchers did not report good results from a major trial testing L-carnitine on Alzheimer's patients. However, since L-carnitine is also excellent for the heart, I see no reason not to use it.

Control Stress • Learning how to cope with stress, and getting help when you are feeling overwhelmed may be the best preventive medicine against Alzheimer's. Several studies have shown that chronic stress can hamper the performance of cells in key parts of the brain, resulting in Alzheimer's-type symptoms such as memory loss and impaired mental capabilities. The damage occurs in the hippocampus, the portion of the brain essential for memory and learning. In animal studies, researchers have proven that prolonged stress can increase the signs of aging in the brain, and many suspect that the same may be true for humans. During stressful situations, people produce cortisol, a stress hormone that revs the body up, giving them the physical and mental stamina to withstand the extra pressure. Researchers at McGill University recently found that people with higher levels of stress hormones in their blood did not perform as well on tests of attention and memory as people with lower levels. In fact, older people with lower levels of stress hormones fared just as well as young people in cognitive tests, while those with higher stress hormone levels got scores up to 50 percent lower.

Some researchers believe that people become more susceptible to the ill effects of stress hormones as they age. In some cases, people may produce too much stress hormone, which could cause damage to brain cells. Interestingly, stress hormone levels have been found to be higher and more difficult to control in Alzheimer's patients.

A Word About Estrogen • Some studies have found that hormone replacement therapy may help prevent Alzheimer's disease in women. For example, researchers at the University of Southern California have found that women who take estrogen replacement therapy after menopause cut their risk of getting Alzheimer's disease by more than 40 percent, and if they do get it, they have much less severe symptoms. Other studies have shown that estrogen can increase the growth of dendrites and triggers the production of choline acetyltransferase, an enzyme that helps carry signals among neurons. However, before popping an estrogen pill, keep in mind that another major California study has found that estrogen has little, if any, effect on the incidence or course of Alzheimer's. In addition, estrogen replacement therapy is not without risk; women who take estrogen increase the odds of getting cancers of the breast and uterus. In addition, estrogen can be dangerous for women with certain medical conditions, including high blood pressure, clotting problems, and migraine headaches.

Garlic • French researchers recently reported that aged garlic extract appeared to slow down brain deterioration in aged laboratory rats with an Alzheimer's-type disease. In addition, the garlic normalized the brain's serotonin system; if the serotinin system malfunctions, it can cause depression. Although we don't know whether garlic will work as well on human brains, I feel that since garlic offers so many other benefits, it is wise to include it in your daily diet or take a garlic supplement.

Arthritis

Arthritis, which literally means the inflammation of a joint, is a general term used to described about 125 different conditions. The term *arthritis* encompasses a wide range of ailments ranging from osteoarthritis, the so-called wear and tear arthritis associated with advanced age, to gout, a painful condition caused by high blood levels of uric acid, to lupus, an autoimmune disease that primarily affects women. Due to the aging of the population, arthritis is a growing problem in the United States. According to a recent study by the Centers for Disease Control and Prevention, by the year 2020, nearly one in five Americans will suffer from some form of arthritic disease (as compared to one out of six today).

In this section, I will talk about the two most common forms of arthritis: osteoarthritis and rheumatoid arthritis.

Osteoarthritis

Also known as *degenerative joint disease,* osteoarthritis affects about 16 million Americans and usually strikes after age forty-five. Osteoarthritis is characterized by swollen joints, achiness, and stiffness or pain in the hands, spine, hips, or knees. It is caused by a gradual wearing away of the cartilage, the sponge-like material that cushions the ends of the bones, preventing them from rubbing together. In some cases, an injury to a bone or joint will cause osteoarthritic changes.

Bone X rays of most people over fifty will show some signs of osteoarthritis, and although it can cause some discomfort, it is rarely crippling. In fact, researchers suspect that people with severe osteoarthritis may have a genetic form of the disease. There is no cure for osteoarthritis; as of yet, we don't know how to stimulate the body to regenerate cartilage. And for most people, aspirin or its herbal counterpart, white willow bark, or acetaminophen may be all that's needed to control the occasional bouts of pain. However, there are several things that people can do to prevent osteoporosis from becoming a problem.

EARL'S RX

Lighten Up   •   The knee is typically the first area in the body to be affected by osteoarthritis, which in severe cases can impair mobility. Numerous studies have shown that overweight people are at greater risk of developing arthritic knees than normal-weight people.

Get Physical   •   Exercise may be the best preventive medicine against developing arthritis. Researchers suspect that exercise may help to retain cartilage by increasing the flow of blood to knee joints and other crucial areas, which is necessary to nourish cells. Walking, swimming, cycling, and rowing are excellent choices for most people because they move joints in a safe way. Sports such as tennis, basketball, and soccer, which require pivoting and sudden moves, may be riskier in terms of injury. Contrary to common belief, even a high-impact aerobic exercise such as running may be beneficial (but only for people who do not have osteoarthritis). Researchers at Stanford University studied the knee X rays of fifty men and women who ran about 3 hours a week. Some members of the study decreased their activity while others increased or maintained their time running. At the end of 2 years, researchers did not find any problems in the X rays of the most active group that would suggest that running had worn down cartilage.

At one time, people with osteoarthritis were advised to avoid the stress and strain of exercise. We now know that was precisely the wrong advice. For example, in a study conducted at the Hospital for Special Surgery and Columbia University, researchers found that people with osteoarthritis of the knee who followed a supervised walking program experienced improved mobility and decreased pain as compared to those who remained inactive. However, osteoarthritis sufferers should beware of any activity that further stresses already vulnerable knee and ankle joints. Running, jogging, and sports that require a lot of pivoting, such as skiing and basketball, may cause more harm than good. So what's left? According to the Arthritis Foundation, the solution may lie to the East: tai chi, a form of martial arts based on gentle, flowing movements, can provide a good workout without overworking the joints. In fact, the Arthritis Foundation is offering classes in tai chi. For more information on safe ways to exercise, call the national office (800-283-7800) or your local chapter.

Avoid Injuries • Warm up before exercising; warmed-up joints are less likely to be injured. Stretching limbers up muscles and tendons and improves joint mobility; in other words, it primes you for your workout. Take a stretch and tone class at your local Y or consult with a sports medicine specialist. Most importantly, don't overexert yourself if you're tired—that's likely to make you accident prone.

Become safety conscious. A little thought ahead of time can help to avert common injuries such as slipping on ice in the winter or falling in the tub that can damage cartilate and begin a downward spiral of pain and inactivity. Wear solid low-heeled boots or shoes outdoors. Be sure that your bathroom is designed for safety—more falls occur in the bathroom than anywhere else in the house. Repair lose or broken steps or anything else around the house or workplace that could promote injury.

Dietary Tips • Some people find that certain foods may aggravate their arthritis. Obviously, if you consistently feel worse after eating a particular food, try eliminating it from your diet and see if you improve. In addition, some people may find the nightshade vegetables (e.g., potatoes, tomatoes, peppers, and eggplants) to be irritating.

Antioxidants • Some researchers believe that degenerative diseases such as arthritis are caused by damage inflicted by free radicals, highly unstable oxygen molecules that can, among other things, promote premature aging. A daily antioxidant supplement including vitamins and minerals such as beta-carotene, vitamins C and E, and selenium may help to prevent or slow down arthritic changes.

Herbal Remedies

Ashwaganda • Part of the traditional Indian system of medicine called Ayurvedic, ashwaganda has been shown to reduce pain and stiffness caused by osteoarthritis. Ahwaganda is sold in natural food stores in tea and capsule form.

Boswellin Cream • Also from the Ayurvedic healing tradition, this greaseless cream contains extracts of *Boswellia serrata* plant, vitamin E, capsaicin, and methyl salicylate.

Cayenne Creams and Ointments • Creams and ointments containing cayenne pepper can help reduce pain by stimulating the production of endorphins, the body's own natural painkiller. Many are sold over the counter at drug and natural food stores.

Licorice • This herb stimulates the production of two steroids: cortisone and aldosterone, which can help relieve pain and inflammation (Aldosterone raises blood pressure; therefore, licorice should not be used by people with high blood pressure.) Licorice is available in tea and capsule form.

Rheumatoid Arthritis

About 2.1 million people in the United States—two-thirds of them women—suffer from rheumatoid arthritis, a condition that causes painful inflammation in the joints and can result in severe disability. Unlike osteoarthritis (which is caused by the wearing away of cartilage), rheumatoid arthritis is characterized by a glitch in the immune system that causes it to attack the collagen, which lines the membranes of the joint. No one knows the cause of rheumatoid arthritis, although some researchers suspect that an initial infection may be responsible for throwing the immune system out of whack, which triggers the autoimmune reaction. In addition, there appears to be a genetic tendency to develop rheumatoid arthritis. Although rheumatoid arthritis can strike young women, most cases of rheumatoid arthritis occur between ages forty and sixty.

If you have rheumatoid arthritis, you should be under the care of a physician or knowledgeable natural healer. Although there is no cure, there are many treatments available today that can help relieve pain and discomfort. In addition to conventional treatments, which range from anti-inflammatory medications such as aspirin or ibuprofin to antibiotics to immunosuppressor drugs, here are some alternative treatments that may help.

EARL'S RX

Gamma-linolenic Acid • Gamma-linolenic acid (GLA), which is found in evening primrose oil and borage seed oil, is an omega-6 fatty acid that is similar to the omega-3 fatty acids found in fatty fish. Natural healers have long prescribed evening primrose oil to treat rheumatoid arthritis. A recent study performed at the University of Pennsylvania found that a daily dose of 1.4 grams of GLA could significantly reduce symptoms such as pain and joint swelling in patients with rheumatoid arthritis. Capsules of evening primrose oil and borage seed oil are available at natural food stores.

Omega-3 Fatty Acids • Several studies have confirmed that many people with rheumatoid arthritis have shown improvement after taking supplements of omega-3 fatty acids. Omega-3 fatty acids contain compounds that can inhibit the inflammatory response in the body.

Chicken Cartilage • Chew on some chicken bones! According to a study performed at Boston's Beth Israel Hospital, chicken cartilage protein, which is found in chicken bones, can help relieve the symptoms of rheumatoid arthritis. In the study, one group of patients drank a solution made from chicken collagen in a glass of orange juice daily, whereas the other group drank a placebo. Out of the chicken collagen group, four patients went into complete remission, and the others had a significant reduction in symptoms. In the placebo group, however, none of the patients went into remission, although a small group (four out of thirty-one) said they felt better, which researchers attributed to the "placebo effect."

Dietary Tips • There is also some evidence that a low-fat diet may help to relieve symptoms such as pain and stiffness. In a study conducted by Loma Linda University in California, rheumatoid arthritis patients were given instructions on diet and stress reduction several times weekly for a 5-week period. The participants cut their daily calories by about 30 percent and reduced their fat intake to about 10 percent of their daily caloric intake. After 3 months, the group experienced vast improvement in the amount of stiffness and discomfort.

Other studies have shown that arthritis sufferers who eat a vegetarian diet can find relief from their discomfort. Researchers can't say whether meat actually contributes to arthritic flares or whether it's the increased intake of fruits and vegetables that alleviates the symptoms.

Some rheumatoid arthritis patients have found that certain

foods may trigger a flare, and studies confirm that rheumatoid patients often develop allergic reactions to many foods. According to recent studies, rheumatoid patients often show signs of sensitivity to foods such as corn, wheat, bacon, oranges, milk, and oats. However, researchers are not sure whether food sensitivities actually contribute to arthritis. Eliminating dairy products and nightshade vegetables such as tomatoes, potatoes, bell peppers, tobacco, and eggplant may help your condition.

Herbal Remedies   •

Horsetail   •   This herb contains minute quantities of gold, which may be effective against joint pain and stiffness. It is sold in tea and capsule form in natural food stores.

Propolis   •   Found in honey, this substance blocks enzymes that produce prostaglandins, hormonelike substances that can cause pain and inflammation. Propolis is sold in natural food stores.

Turmeric   •   This herb, which is used in curry powder, is a natural anti-inflammatory.

Wild Yam   •   This herb contains steroidal compounds that have an anti-inflammatory effect. It is available in tea and capsule form and is used in many herbal arthritis formulas.

Yucca   •   This native American herb is a long-time favorite for treating rheumatoid arthritis and is sold in natural food stores in tea and capsule form.

Cataracts

A cataract is a cloudy or opaque covering that grows over the lens of the eye, which can cause partial or total blindness. In rare cases, cataracts may be due to a genetic problem. In most cases, however, cataracts are a result of cellular damage to the eye lens inflicted by ultraviolet light or oxidation. Cataracts are very common among older people; it is estimated that as many as 50 million people worldwide are cataract sufferers. In fact, in the United States alone, over 1 million surgeries are performed each year to remove cataracts. According to the Nutrition and Cataract Research Laboratory at Tufts University, if we could postpone the formation of cataracts by 10 years, the United States could save more than $1.5 billion annually.

EARL'S RX

Cover Your Eyes • To protect against ultraviolet (UV) light, wear sunglasses outdoors, not just in the summer, but all year long. Be sure to buy sunglasses that specifically promise to block 99 to 100 percent of UVA and UVB rays. Not all sunglasses are effective; check with your eye doctor to see which glasses are right for you. In addition, a hat with a wide brim can block about 50 percent of UV light. (It can also help prevent wrinkles.)

Needless to say, avoid unnecessary exposure to UV light, such as tanning salons (which may also promote skin cancer).

Eat Your Fruits and Vegetables • According to researchers at the Human Nutrition Research Center at Tufts University, older adults with cataracts reported eating significantly fewer servings of fruits and vegetables than those who were cataract free. In fact, those who ate fewer than three and a half servings of fruits and vegetables daily had a fivefold greater risk of developing senile cataracts than people who ate more. This is not surprising, considering the fact that other studies have shown that people with cataracts have lower blood levels of carotenoids and vitamin C, compounds that are abundant in fruits and vegetables.

Take Your Vitamins • Antioxidants such as vitamin C, beta-carotene, and vitamin E may help prevent against oxidative damage that can lead to the formation of cataracts. For example, in one study performed at the U.S. Department of Agriculture's Human Nutrition Center on Aging at Tufts University, when vitamin C was added to the diets of guinea pigs, their eyes showed less oxidative damage after exposure to UV light than pigs who were not given the vitamin.

Other vitamins and minerals may also play a role in preventing cataracts. In a landmark study conducted by the National Eye Institute and the Chinese Academy of Medicine in Beijing, researchers gave more than 2100 Chinese adults (ages forty-five to seventy-four) in a malnourished population of Linxian either 2 Centrum multivitamin and mineral tablets and 25,000 international units of beta-carotene daily or a placebo. After 5 years, the vitamin takers were 43 percent less likely to have nuclear cataracts (cataracts that form in the center of the eye) than the placebo group.

In a second test, more than 3200 Linxian residents were given 2.3 milligrams of riboflavin and 40 milligrams of niacin daily. After 5 years, those who took the vitamins were 50 percent less likely to develop nuclear cataracts than those who didn't take the vitamins. Researchers speculate that riboflavin may have helped prevent cataracts because it is involved in the production of glutathione, a potent antioxidant in the eye lens.

Coronary Artery Disease

Heart disease is a national epidemic—it is the number one killer of men and women in the United States. When we talk about heart disease, we're really talking about coronary artery disease (CAD), a condition in which the arteries bringing blood to the heart become clogged or obstructed with a yellowish, waxy substance called *plaque* (the condition is known as *atherosclerosis*). If the arteries become too narrow, the flow of blood and oxygen to the heart will become severely impaired, which can lead to a heart attack.

Some people are more CAD-prone than others due to such factors as age, genetics, or lifestyle. The risk of developing CAD increases with age; about 55 percent of all heart attacks occur after age fifty-five. Before age fifty-five, men have a higher rate of heart disease, but postmenopausal women quickly catch up to men. Race is another risk factor. African-Americans have a higher rate of CAD than whites. People with a parent or sibling who has had a heart attack before age fifty-five (age sixty-five for women) are automatically put in a higher risk group for CAD. And in addition to immutable risk factors such as sex, age, and race, there are other more controllable risk factors that are equally important, including smoking, obesity, sedentary lifestyle, diabetes, high blood pressure, and high blood cholesterol levels. Few people are risk free. In fact, according to a recent study by the Centers for Disease Control and Prevention, more than 80 percent of all American adults have one or more risk factors for CAD. But take heart—even if you have one or more risk factors, it doesn't mean that you're going to have a heart attack. Although you may have no control over your genes or your race, you can control many of the other risk factors and, by doing so, can dramatically reduce the odds of developing CAD.

EARL'S RX

Caution: If you have a heart condition or are taking medicine for a heart problem, do not use any herbs, drugs, or supplements without first checking with your physician or natural healer.

Up in Smoke • Up to 40 percent of CAD deaths each year are believed to be due to smoke-related problems. Given the fact that smoking has also been associated with an increased risk of developing many different forms of cancer, by now, even the Marlboro Man knows that it's time to "butt out." But what you may not know is that secondhand smoke from someone else's cigarette may be inflicting damage to *your* heart. Researchers at New York University Medical Center have shown that exposure to secondhand smoke can accelerate the formation of plaque deposits in the arteries of male chicks. In fact, according to the study, the smoke-exposed chicks had plaques that were significantly larger than non-smoke-exposed chicks. Although no one knows whether human arteries behave quite the same way, it makes good sense to reduce your exposure to cigarette smoke.

Hold the Hostility • According to researchers at the National Institute on Aging and the University of Maryland, angry, hostile people are at greater risk of developing heart disease, especially if "they are arrogant, argumentative, surly, and rude." My hunch is that these people are also carriers, inflicting damage on their families and anyone else they come in contact with. If you find yourself losing control, seek professional help.

Know Your Numbers • Blood cholesterol levels should be maintained at under 200 milligrams per deciliter. High-density lipoproteins (HDLs) or "good" cholesterol, should be 35 or above. The low-density lipoproteins (LDLs): HDLs ratio should be 3:1 but should never dip below 4:1. For example, if the LDL level is 120, then HDLs should be 40. Eating a diet in which less than 25 percent of your daily calories is derived from fat will help maintain a low cholesterol. In addition, watch your intake of saturated fat (primarily from animal products) and polyunsaturated fat from foods such as margarine, which contain *trans*-fatty acids that can raise blood cholesterol levels.

Foods that are rich in fiber, including oat bran, psyllium, and pectin, which is found in grapefruit, can help lower total cholesterol.

Keep track of another type of blood lipid: triglycerides. Elevated levels of triglycerides are a risk factor for heart disease. Women should maintain triglyceride levels under 200 milligrams per deciliter, and men should maintain levels under 400 miligrams per deciliter.

Boost Your HDLs • If your HDLs are low, there are some things that you can do to raise them:

- Exercise has been shown to raise HDLs, especially if you've been sedentary. A 2-mile walk four or five times a week at a moderately brisk pace may bring your HDLs up to speed.

- A glass of red wine daily has been shown to raise HDLs.
- An onion a day can raise your HDLs.
- Niacin (100 milligrams daily) taken with chromium (600 micrograms daily) can lower cholesterol and raise HDLs. (High doses of niacin can be toxic to your liver and should be taken only under the supervision of a physician.)
- Eating four or five smaller meals frequently throughout the day instead of the usual "three squares" has been shown to lower cholesterol and increase HDLs.

Take Your Antioxidants • Several studies have shown that people who take antioxidant supplements have lower rates of heart disease than people who don't. Antioxidants such as vitamin C, beta-carotene, vitamin E, and selenium help prevent the oxidation of LDL cholesterol, which is believed to contribute to the formation of plaque.

Many herbs, including basil, dill, mint, parsley, and rosemary, are excellent sources of antioxidants.

Aspirin • A recent study of 22,000 male doctors showed that those who took 325 milligrams of aspirin daily (the amount in one adult aspirin) had 44 percent fewer heart attacks than those who didn't. Talk to your physician or natural healer before using aspirin on a regular basis.

Pass on the Sugar • The American diet is high in sugary foods, and this may contribute to the high incidence of heart disease. According to a recent study, high levels of dietary fructose, a sweetener derived from corn that is a common ingredient in foods, can raise blood serum LDL levels. Ironically, many of the new low-fat or no fat-baked products on the market include fructose. Consume these foods in moderation.

Those Amazing Monos • People in Mediterranean countries eat a diet rich in monounsaturated fats (mostly from olive oil) and not so coincidentally have the lowest rates of heart disease in the world. Studies have shown that monounsaturated fats can reduce overall blood cholesterol and specifically can cut LDL cholesterol.

Monounsaturated fats combined with vitamin E may be a particularly potent way to attack LDLs. Researchers from the University of California, San Diego, La Jolla discovered that oleic acid (which is found in monounsaturated fat) and vitamin E prevented the oxidation of a particular type of LDL—the smallest, densest portion of the LDL particle. Studies have shown that the small, dense LDL is more susceptible to oxidative damage than the larger LDL particle. About 33 percent of all men and 15 percent of all women have LDLs that are predominantly small and dense and thus may be at greater risk of developing CAD. In the California study, eighteen healthy volunteers (nine men and nine women, ages twenty-two to sixty-one) were given 1200 milligrams daily of vitamin E. Six of the eighteen volunteers ate the normal American diet, which is high in saturated fats; six ate a diet high in polyunsaturated fats; and six ate a diet high in oleic acids. Blood samples from the three groups showed that the rates of LDL oxidation for both dense and larger LDL particles were lowest in the oleic-enriched group.

Omega-3 Fatty Acids • Found in fatty fish, omega-3 fatty acids have been shown to decrease blood cholesterol and triglycerides. Omega-3 fatty acids can also help prevent blood clots. Good sources include mackerel, salmon, albacore tuna, herring, and lake trout. Fish oil capsules are available at natural food stores.

Herbal Remedies • Several herbs can help prevent heart disease.

Capsaicin • Capsaicin from hot chilies can lower blood triglyceride levels. Pour on the hot sauce!

Gamma-linolenic Acid • Gamma-linolenic acid, which is found in borage oil and evening primrose oil, is an effective cholesterol-lowering agent.

Ginger • Ginger can help prevent the formation of blood clots, which can lead to a heart attack.

Ginseng • Ginseng can help lower cholesterol.

Green Tea • Several animal studies confirm that compounds in green tea called *catechins* can lower cholesterol. Not so coincidentally, Japanese men have the lowest rate of heart disease in the world, and Japanese women have the second lowest rate (second only to France).

Hawthorn • This herb has been used for centuries in Europe to treat heart ailments. Hawthorn is rich in bioflavonoids, which can help strengthen tiny blood vessels called *capillaries*, thus improving the flow of blood throughout the body. Animal studies have shown that this herb can increase the contractility of the heart muscle, strengthening the heart's ability to pump blood. In fact, in Europe, hawthorn may be prescribed along with the drug digitalis to regulate the heartbeat.

Oriental Mushrooms • Reishi and shiitake mushrooms can lower cholesterol and prevent blood clots.

Turmeric • This spice, which is used in curry powder, is a natural blood thinner.

Other Supplements

Coenzyme Q10 • Coenzyme Q_{10} is found in every cell in the body, and as we age, levels of this enzyme begin to fall off. Coenzyme Q_{10} helps facilitate the process that provides energy to cells and improves the circulation of blood. In Japan, Coenzyme Q_{10} is used to treat angina, chest pain caused by a diminished blood supply due to CAD. Coenzyme Q_{10} capsules and tablets are sold at natural food stores. I recommend 30 milligrams daily.

L-Carnitine • L-Carnitine is a nonprotein amino acid that is found in the heart and skeletal muscle and helps to carry fatty acids across the mitochondria of the cell, thus providing heart and skeletal cells with energy. Some researchers believe that a deficiency of this amino acid may increase the risk of having a heart attack. Studies have shown that L-carnitine can also lower cholesterol and triglyceride levels and raise HDLs. L-Carnitine capsules are sold at natural food stores. I recommend 1 gram (1000 milligrams) daily.

Colorectal Cancer

About fifty thousand Americans die of colorectal cancer (cancer of either the colon or the rectum) each year, making it the third leading cause of cancer deaths. Each year, about 160,000 new cases are diagnosed. About 10 percent of all cases of colorectal cancer are genetic: as of this writing, geneticists have identified at least two genes that are believed to be responsible for this disease and even more may be involved. However, more researchers believe that perhaps as many as 90 percent of all colorectal cancers may be due to environmental factors, such as diet and lifestyle. Although colorectal cancer is common in the West, it is rare in the third world.

The warning signs include rectal bleeding, blood in the stool, and a change in bowel habits. (If you experience any of these symptoms, contact your physician for further tests.)

EARL'S RX

Cut the Fat • A high-fat diet can indirectly promote the growth of tumors in the colon. During digestion, fat stimulates the release of bile acids by the gallbladder. The fat and bile then travel through the small intestine to the colon. In the colon, the bile is converted into chemicals called *secondary bile acids*, which over time can produce cancerous changes in the colon. The less fat consumed, the smaller the amount of bile that is produced, resulting in a smaller amount of potentially carcinogenic secondary bile acids.

Wheat Bran • Researchers have known for some time that a high-fiber diet appears to protect against colon cancer. However, recent studies suggest that wheat bran may be one of the most potent protectors. A study conducted at the American Health Foundation in Valhalla, New York, compared the effects of different dietary fibers on seventy-eight women. Each of the women ate three or four muffins daily containing either corn, oat, or wheat bran for 2 months (consuming about 30 grams of fiber daily). At the end of the study, researchers measured the level of tumor-promoting enzymes and bile acids in the intestinal tract of the volunteers and found that only the wheat bran decreased the concentration of these potentially hazardous compounds.

In another recent study at New York Hospital/Cornell Medical Center, fifty-eight people with precancerous polyps were divided into two groups. One group was put on a high-fiber diet rich in wheat bran cereal and the other group was given a low-fiber cereal. Most of the people eating the wheat bran experienced a reduction in the size and number of their polyps. There was no change seen in those on the low-fiber diet.

Eat Your Five a Day • A major 6-year study of the diets of more than 764,000 adults by the National Cancer Institute and the American Cancer Society confirmed that those who consumed the least amount of fruits and vegetables were the most likely to develop colon cancer.

Protease Inhibitors • Compounds found in legumes called *protease inhibitors* may help to prevent colon cancer. For example, soybeans contain a unique protease inhibitor: the Bowman–Birk inhibitor, which has been shown to stop the spread of many different forms of cancer, including colon cancer. For example, in rats fed a carcinogen known to induce colon cancer, adding Bowman–Birk inhibitor concentrate to their diet suppressed the formation of tumors in 100 percent of the animals.

Indoles • Indoles are compounds found in cruciferous vegetables including bok choy (Chinese cabbage), broccoli, cauliflower, and brussels sprouts. Some studies suggest that indoles may help prevent cancerous changes in the colon.

Aspirin • Based on a study of more than 635,000 people performed by the American Cancer Society, those who took aspirin were at significantly lower risk of dying from colon cancer. In fact, men and women who took aspirin at least sixteen times a month were 40 percent less likely to die from cancers of the digestive tract than those who did not. Talk to your physician about whether or not you should take aspirin.

Calcium and Vitamin D • Several studies have found a link between low calcium/vitamin D consumption and an increased risk of colorectal cancer. A major 19-year population study of more than 25,000 people in Chicago found that those who had an average daily intake of 1200 milligrams of calcium daily had a 50 percent reduced risk of the disease. Researchers suspect that calcium may bind with bile, thus preventing it from irritating the colon wall.

Exercise • A sedentary lifestyle has been linked to an increased risk of colorectal cancer. In one study, men who scored the lowest in terms of activity had nearly twice the risk of colorectal cancer as the most active men. Presumably, the same is true for women.

Constipation

Constipation is a very common problem among older adults. As we age, the digestive system slows down a bit, making it harder to break down food and eliminate waste. In addition, hormonal changes during menopause can cause occasional bouts of constipation in some women. And prescription drugs such as diuretics, painkillers, tranquilizers, and even antihistamines can promote constipation. However, very often diet and lifestyle are the main culprits, and making simple changes can help to keep you regular.

EARL'S RX

Exercise • I think that inactivity is one of the main reasons why older people (and many younger ones) suffer from constipation. Sitting at a desk all day or sitting in your car prevents your body from working well. You don't have to overdo it; a simple walking program could make a real difference.

Water • Drinking 8 to 10 glasses of filtered water per day will help to increase intestinal motility and prevent constipation.

Fiber • Insoluble fiber—the kind found in foods such as celery, wheat bran, legumes, and most fruits and vegetables—softens and bulks waste to help move it more quickly through the colon, thus helping to prevent constipation. Try to eat between 20 and 30 grams of fiber daily. However, it may not always be easy to get enough fiber from food alone. Therefore, I recommend taking *psyllium* daily. Simply add a teaspoon of psyllium to water or juice, and follow with 2 glasses of water. (**Caution: Psyllium can cause allergic reactions in some people. If you are allergic to different foods, check with your allergy specialist before using psyllium.**)

To prevent bloating and gas, add more fiber to your diet slowly: if you have a low intake of fiber, don't shock your system by dumping in the whole 30 grams in 1 day. Give yourself time to get used to the new foods. If you have a bowel disorder, check with your physician before adding fiber to your diet.

Diabetes

More than 14 million Americans have diabetes, a disease characterized by an excess amount of sugar in the blood and urine. Juvenile diabetes, which occurs during childhood, is caused by the failure of the pancreas to produce enough *insulin,* the hormone that breaks down glucose or sugar so that it can be utilized by body cells. Adult-onset diabetes is somewhat different. In this case, the body produces enough insulin; however, the insulin works less efficiently. The precise cause of diabetes is still unknown; however, in some cases, it may be triggered by a viral infection. There also appears to be a strong genetic component.

Most people don't think of diabetes as a disease of aging, but that's precisely what it is. Eighty-five percent of all cases of diabetes occur in people ages thirty-five and older. If untreated, diabetes can lead to serious complications including heart disease, kidney disease, stroke, and severe circulatory problems. Many diabetics require insulin shots and/or medication that stimulates the production of insulin by the pancreas. However, many diabetics are treated solely through dietary regulation and the careful monitoring of blood and urine sugar.

About one in four Americans have a genetic tendency to develop adult diabetes. Women are twice as likely to develop diabetes as men. However, there is strong evidence that a proper diet and lifestyle can prevent or delay the onset of diabetes.

EARL'S RX

Stay Trim • Obesity is a major risk factor for diabetes (as well as a host of other diseases including coronary artery disease, stroke, and several forms of cancer). Insulin is produced by special cells in the pancreas called beta cells. Beta cells in the pancreas manufacture and store insulin until a rising blood sugar level signals to them to release them. Over time, however, beta cells begin to wear out. It stands to reason that people who consume large quantities of food—especially sugar—may be using up their life's supply of beta cells quicker than others who consume smaller amounts of food.

High-Fiber Diet • Fiber-rich foods help lower insulin needs. A diet rich in legumes, whole grains, fruits, and vegetables may be your best defense against diabetes (and many other degenerative diseases).

Low-Fat Diet • A high-fat diet appears to hasten the risk of developing diabetes. In one study performed at the University of Colorado Health Sciences Center in Denver, researchers tracked the progress of 123 people with a impaired glucose tolerance, a condition that dramatically increases the risk of developing diabetes. The researchers found that people who ate the diets highest in fat were much more likely to develop diabetes than those who adhered to low-fat diets. In addition, in subsequent blood tests, people eating the lowest amount of fat had normal blood sugar levels.

Monunsaturated Fat • Recent studies suggest that increasing your intake of monounsaturated fat (found in olive oil, canola oil, and avocados) may help stabilize blood sugar levels. Substitute other forms of fat, such as saturated and polyunsaturated, with monounsaturates. Do not exceed 25 percent of your daily calories in the form of any fat.

Exercise • A study performed at the U.S. Department of Agriculture's Human Nutrition Research Center on Aging at Tufts University showed that regular aerobic exercise can lower people's risk of diabetes. Researchers studied eighteen older men and women who had above-normal glucose levels on a glucose tolerance test, which increases their risk of developing diabetes by tenfold. After 12 weeks of cycling on an ergometer 4 days per week, the eighteen volunteers increased their blood glucose clearance by 11 percent. In addition, the exercise appeared to improve the ability of their cells to respond to insulin.

Supplements

Chromium • Animal studies have shown that chromium, a trace mineral, can help the body use insulin more efficiently; therefore, less insulin is required to break down sugar. Human studies have confirmed that chromium can reduce blood sugar levels in people with elevated blood sugar. Chromium is found in broccoli, cheese, brewer's yeast, shellfish, and whole wheat English muffins. Chromium supplements are sold in natural food stores. Take 200 micrograms daily.

Magnesium • Older people often become insulin resistant, that is, their insulin does not work as efficiently as it should. Insulin resistance increases the risk of developing diabetes. Studies show that magnesium supplements can help older people improve their ability to metabolize glucose.

Vitamin E (Tocopherol) • A recent Italian study showed that daily Vitamin E supplements of 900 milligrams for four months helped people with adult-onset diabetes use insulin more efficiently, thus helping to normalize blood sugar levels.

Herbal Remedies • U.S. Department of Agriculture researchers used a test-tube assay of insulin activity to identify plants that may help prevent diabetes. Nine plants were found to improve insulin activity including sage, lavender, bearberry (*Uva ursi*), hops, and oregano. (All these herbs and spices are available in natural food stores.) Other potential herbal remedies for diabetes include the following:

Cinnamon • In test tube studies, this spice appeared to significantly increase the ability of insulin to metabolize glucose. Take 1 to 3 capsules daily or sprinkle 1 to 2 tablespoons of cinnamon on your cereal.

Fenugreek • Fenugreek seeds (used to flavor curry and chutney) contain many different compounds that can help prevent surges in blood sugar. Take 1 to 3 capsules daily.

Garlic • Sauté some garlic in that olive oil! Garlic contains an amino acid called *S*-allylcysteine sulfoxide, which in animal studies has been shown to significantly decrease blood sugar and cholesterol levels. Garlic is also available in tablets and capsule form. Follow the package directions.

Turmeric • The spice that gives curry its golden color, turmeric has been shown to enhance the activity of insulin in test tube studies. Take 1 to 3 capsules daily.

Digestive Disorders

As we age, our bodies produce less hydrochloric acid, which is essential for the digestion of food, especially fibrous meats, vegetables, and poultry. As a result, it is quite common for people over fifty to develop chronic indigestion, which is characterized by gas and bloating after eating. Typically, people with this problem self-medicate by popping over-the-counter antacids. However, that is precisely the wrong treatment, because antacids actually reduce the amount of acid. Thus, the problem worsens. If you have chronic indigestion, first check with your physician or natural healer for an accurate diagnosis: the symptoms could also be related to an ulcer or other medical problem. If your symptoms are due to a reduction in HCl, try the following natural remedies.

EARL'S RX

Eat Smaller Meals • Smaller, lighter meals are kinder on the digestive system than larger, heavier meals. Try to eat small amounts of lean meat, fish, or poultry accompanied by lightly cooked vegetables.

Digestive Aids • There are several over-the-counter digestive aids sold in natural food stores that may help break down food. *Bromelain* is an enzyme found in pineapple that can help digest food and absorb vitamins. It is often used with *papain,* an enzyme found in papaya that can help break down proteins. Both are sold at natural food stores in a chewable tablet form. Chew one 500-milligram tablet daily.

   Betaine hydrochloric acid (made from beets) can also help to get the digestive juices flowing. Take one or two 500-milligram tablets with food up to three times daily.

Herbal Teas • Several herbal teas are excellent for digestion problems. Anise, fennel, and peppermint teas (all sold at natural food stores) are particularly soothing for an agitated stomach.

Diverticulosis

Diverticulosis is a condition characterized by the formation of tiny pouches, or diverticula, in the wall of the colon. Diverticulosis is rare among children and young adults but quite common among people over forty. By age sixty, about half of all people have diverticulosis.

Diverticulosis appears to be a natural part of the aging process and is not serious. However, in rare cases, the diverticula can become inflamed, which can lead to intestinal obstruction. The more serious diverticulitis appears to be related to chronic constipation and straining during bowel movements.

EARL'S RX

Avoid Constipation • A diet rich in fruit, vegetables, and whole grains is usually all it takes to maintain regular bowel habits.

Gallstones

The gallbladder is a sac in which bile from the liver is stored. Bile is essential for proper digestion. Gallstones are solid masses that form in the gallbladder or bile ducts, which can cause inflammation and pain. Up until age fifty, gallstones are more common among women than men; however, at that time, men are equally vulnerable. People with liver disease may be more prone to developing gallstones.

There are three types of gallstones: cholesterol stones, those consisting of pure bile, and stones that are mixtures of bile, cholesterol, and calcium. In some cases, gallstones can be dissolved with drugs, but if not, surgery may be required to remove them. Chronic gallbladder disease may result in the surgical removal of the gallbladder, a cholecystectomy, which is the fifth most common operation performed in the United States each year. However, through diet and supplements, many people can successfully maintain a healthy gallbladder.

EARL'S RX

Low-Fat Diet • An excess amount of fat may result in the overproduction of bile by the liver, which could lead to the formation of gallstones.

Lecithin • Lecithin supplements may help to control cholesterol buildup and may help to prevent gallstones. Lecithin is sold in granule and capsule form at natural food stores. Take 1 tablespoon of the granules or 6 capsules daily.

Herbal Remedies

Dandelion • This herb—or weed, depending on your point of view—enhances liver and gallbladder function and has traditionally been used by herbal healers to treat ailments related to these organs. Interestingly, dandelion is a rich source of lecithin. Eat fresh dandelion in salads, or buy the capsules at natural food stores. Take 1 to 3 capsules daily.

Turmeric • Studies performed in Germany and India show that this spice may help to prevent gallstones, probably by enhancing the action of the liver and gallbladder. Use this spice in cooking or take a 300-milligram capsule up to three times daily.

Gout

Gout is a particularly painful form of arthritis caused by the accumulation of *uric acid*, a substance that is produced by the body from purines, compounds that are found in many different foods. Excess uric acid forms crystallike deposits in joints—typically in the large joint of one or both big toes—which can lead to arthritic-type swelling and pain. More than 2 million Americans suffer from gout; gout is much more common among men than women. After menopause, women are at a higher risk of developing this disease.

Gout tends to run in families. However, in some cases, the condition can be brought on by the use of diuretics and other drugs. Gout can be successfully treated with allopurinol (marketed under the names Lopurin and Zyloprim), which can control the rate at which the body produces uric acid. Other medications can speed up the rate at which the body disposes of uric acid in the urine. Although drug treatment has proven to be quite effective, eating too much of the wrong foods (and drinking too much of the wrong drinks) can still trigger a painful gout attack. If untreated, gout can cause permanent damage to the joints.

EARL'S RX

Watch Your Weight • Being overweight increases the odds of developing gout. Researchers at Johns Hopkins University tracked the health and weight of twelve hundred medical students for three decades. Those who had put on the most weight during early adulthood had a much higher incidence of gout than those who stayed trim.

Watch the Purines • Much of the misery of gout can be prevented by maintaining a sensible diet. People with gout should severely limit their intake of foods rich in purines, including mackerel, brains, anchovies, sardines, shrimp, scallops, and sweetbreads. Talk to your physician or natural healer about the right diet for you.

Watch the Booze • Alcoholic beverages—especially straight up on an empty stomach—can trigger an attack.

Do Drink the Water • Ten to twelve glasses of water daily can help flush the excess uric acid crystals out of the body.

Herbal Remedies • Many herbs have been used to help relieve the symptoms of gout.

Burdock root • This herb has been touted as a "blood purifier" because it can help control uric acid levels. Burdock is available in tea or capsule form at natural food stores.

Juniper Berries • Herbalists have used juniper berries to treat gout. This herb may help to prevent gout by normalizing levels of uric acid. (Ironically juniper berries are also used to make gin.) Juniper berry extract and capsules are available at natural food stores.

Gum Disease

Although Americans are getting fewer cavities thanks to the addition of fluoride in the water, gum disease, which can lead to the loss of teeth, is still very common in the United States. According to the 1985–86 National Adult Dental Health Study, nearly half of all adults had bleeding gums (a sign of inflammation), and 24 percent of all adults and 68 percent of all elderly people had significant periodontal attachments in their mouths, often due to tooth loss. Gum disease is usually caused by the accumulation of bacterial plaque near the gum line, which can cause gums to become inflamed. If the gingivitis progresses, it can destroy connective tissue and bones supporting the teeth. However, tooth loss is not an inevitable part of aging:

in most cases, gum disease can be prevented and teeth can be spared.

EARL'S RX

Oral Hygiene • I have difficulty believing that there are still people who are not flossing their teeth daily. It is one of the best ways to keep gum problems at bay.

Avoid Sugar • Sugar is the breeding ground for bacteria. Limit your sugar intake, and in particular, avoid washing your mouth with sugary drinks. Keep in mind that carbohydrates are converted into sugar in the mouth. Brush or rinse your mouth after eating.

Green Tea • Try washing your meals down with green tea! Green tea contains a compound that has an antibacterial action against *Streptococcus mutans,* the bacteria responsible for tooth decay, which can lead to gum problems.

Supplements

Calcium and Vitamin D • Animal studies show that low calcium intake can result in loss of the bone supporting teeth. Human studies show that Americans fall woefully short on this mineral. Be sure to eat calcium-rich foods or to take a calcium/vitamin D supplement daily.

Folic Acid • In human studies, folic acid supplements resulted in less inflammation of the gums in people with gingivitis. Take 400 micrograms of folic acid daily.

Propolis • Propolis, a by-product of honey, is a rich source of bioflavonoids, naturally occurring substances in food that may help to strengthen tiny blood vessels in the gums, thus helping to prevent injury.

Vitamin C Complex • Vitamin C is required for the formation of collagen in connective tissues and is necessary for the repair and maintenance of all body tissues, including the gums. Vitamin C complex includes several bioflavonoids, including rutin, which has been shown to be especially beneficial for gums. Take 1000 milligrams daily of calcium ascorbate.

Coenzyme Q10 • This works well for gum health. Take 30 to 60 milligrams.

Hearing Loss

Presbycusis, the age-related decline in hearing, can begin at around age twenty, when there is a gradual loss in high-frequency hearing. The loss is usually so subtle that it is hardly noticeable. However, by age sixty, there may be a noticeable loss of middle- and low-frequency hearing, making it more difficult to discern human speech. The extent of hearing loss largely depends on two factors: heredity and exposure to loud noises. However, atherosclerosis can also prevent the flow of blood and nutrients to the ear, which could also cause hearing loss.

EARL'S RX

Safeguarding Your Hearing • The best way to preserve your hearing is to avoid bombarding your ears with loud noises, which can actually cause permanent damage to the middle ear. The level of noise considered to be dangerous is 85 to 90 decibels—normal speech is usually 65 to 70 decibels. If you listen to loud music, work around loud machinery, or use many common items such as a lawn mower or vacuum cleaner, you could be exposing yourself to decibel levels that are unsafe. Impulse noise, such as loud explosions from firearms or firecrackers, are particularly dangerous. If you are in situations where you are exposed to loud noises, be sure to wear protective earplugs. They are sold in drugstores and sporting goods stores.

Hemorrhoids

Hemorrhoids are varicose veins in the anus and rectum. (For a full explanation of varicose veins, see p. 228.) Symptoms include pain and light rectal bleeding. (If you have any rectal bleeding, check with your physician. It could be a sign of a gastrointestinal problem or even colon cancer.)

Chronic constipation, pregnancy, or abdominal straining can cause hemorrhoids. In severe cases, surgery may be necessary. However, this is a problem that can usually be controlled through diet and the judicious use of supplements.

EARL'S RX

Avoid Spicy Foods • Hot pepper can aggravate existing hemorrhoids.

Fiber, Fiber, Fiber • The low-fiber diet typical of most Americans is the major cause of hemorrhoids. A diet rich in fruits, vegetables, and whole grains can help keep your bowels functioning normally, which will prevent the kind of straining that can result in hemorrhoids.

Vitamin E • For quick relief, place some vitamin E oil on a cotton ball or swab and apply to the affected area. (Some people are allergic to vitamin E oil. Be sure to try some oil on a small patch of skin and wait 24 hours. Watch for irritation or burning; if there is none, you can proceed with the treatment.)

Herbal Remedies

Butcher's Broom • A salve made from this herb can be applied directly to hemorrhoids. Butcher's broom products are sold in natural food stores.

Ginkgo • This herb helps to promote good circulation, which may help to prevent varicose veins, including hemorrhoids. Take 1 to 3 capsules daily.

High Blood Pressure

When blood is pumped through the heart, it flows through the large arteries into smaller arteries or arterioles. The walls of the arterioles can expand or contract, thus regulating the blood flow. Blood pressure measures the force of blood against the arterial wall. The top number, called the *systolic pressure*, measures the pressure of the blood flow when the heart is beating. The bottom number, called the *diastolic pressure*, measures the pressure of the blood flow when the heart is at rest. A normal adult blood pressure is around 120/80. High blood pressure is defined as a systolic pressure of 140 or above and a diastolic pressure of 90 or above. However, many studies show that a moderately elevated diastolic pressure (85 plus) may be a sign of a problem down the road.

Untreated high blood pressure is dangerous because it means that the heart is working harder than normal to pump blood, which can damage the heart, arteries, and kidneys. High blood pressure is a major risk factor for both heart attack and stroke.

In most cases, the cause of high blood pressure is a mystery. However, in about 5 percent of all cases, the problem can be attributed to an underlying physical problem such as a congenital heart problem, kidney abnormality, or tumor in the adrenal gland.

In the United States, blood pressure rises steadily with age. Men are more likely to develop high blood pressure at younger ages than women; however, by age sixty-five, women are at greater risk of developing high blood pressure than men. I want to stress that high blood pressure is not an inevitable part of aging. In some parts of the world, blood pressure remains relatively stable from childhood through old age. Many researchers believe that diet and lifestyle play a major role in helping to prevent high blood pressure.

There are numerous drugs that are prescribed to control

high blood pressure. Although most work well, nearly all have some undesirable side effects ranging from excessive fatigue to impotency. However, there are many natural alternatives that may work as well in helping to control high blood pressure or even prevent it from happening in the first place. In addition, in many cases, simple changes in diet and lifestyle can reduce the need for medication.

EARL'S RX

Lose Weight • Being overweight increases the risk of developing high blood pressure. Often, a loss in weight is accompanied by a reduction in blood pressure.

Watch the Salt • Many people are salt sensitive, that is, excessive salt in their diet will cause an increase in blood pressure. The American Heart Association recommends limiting your salt intake to 2500 milligrams per day or 1000 milligrams per 1000 calories. In order to achieve this goal, you should probably not add additional salt to your food and steer clear of restaurants that serve highly salted food.

Exercise • A regular exercise program that requires aerobic activity, such as walking 2 miles daily or swimming laps, can help maintain normal blood pressure. In some cases, it can even lower blood pressure in people with high blood pressure.

Limit Alcohol • Drinking more than 2 ounces daily of an alcoholic beverage can increase the risk of developing high blood pressure.

Load Up on the Fruit • According to a study performed at Harvard Medical School, eating a diet high in fruit fiber can help prevent high blood pressure. In their study, the researchers tracked the diets of more than thirty thousand men and found that those who ate less than 12 grams of fruit fiber daily were 60 percent more likely to develop high blood pressure. The researchers found that fruit fiber was more effective in preventing high blood pressure than fiber from grains. Keep in mind, it may not be just the fiber that has a protective effect. Fruit also contains many different compounds, including some that may help to lower blood pressure.

L-Carnitine • L-Carnitine is a nonprotein amino acid found in the heart and skeletal muscle and has been shown to improve the flow of blood to the heart and reduce blood pressure. L-Carnitine is sold at natural food stores.

Mind Your Minerals

Calcium • A 13-year California study of more than 6600 men and women found that people who consumed 1000 milligrams of calcium daily reduced their risk of developing high blood pressure by 20 percent.

Garlic • Aged odorless garlic supplements can lower high blood pressure. Take 3 capsules daily.

Magnesium • A recent study sponsored by the Netherlands Heart Foundation showed that magnesium supplements were effective in controlling high blood pressure in women with mildly high blood pressure who were not on other medication. Six months of magnesium supplementation reduced the systolic pressure by an average of 2.7 and the diastolic pressure by an average of 3.4. Good food sources of magnesium include legumes, green leafy vegetables, whole grains, bananas, low-fat milk, and apricots.

Potassium • Several studies have shown that potassium can help reduce blood pressure. In fact, in one study of fifty-four patients with high blood pressure who were on medication, half the group was given information on increasing their dietary intake of potassium, and the other half was told to continue on their normal diet. At the end of the study, those patients eating the most potassium-rich foods required the least amount of medication to control their blood pressure. In addition, the patients eating the potassium-rich diet felt better and had fewer symptoms. Good sources of potassium include white potatoes, dried apricots, bananas, low-fat yogurt, and oranges.

Herbal Remedies

Astralagus • This herb, which is widely used in China, has been shown to lower blood pressure in animal studies. Astralagus capsules are available in natural food stores and herb shops.

Celery • Researchers at the University of Chicago discovered a compound in celery called 3-butylphthalide that can reduce high blood pressure in laboratory rats. Interestingly, celery is used by Asian healers to treat high blood pressure.

Dong Quai • Studies have shown that this Chinese herb can lower blood pressure in both men and women. Dong Quai is available at natural food stores in tea and capsule form.

Hawthorn • Human and animal studies have shown that hawthorn, a well-known cardiotonic, can reduce blood pressure during exertion. Hawthorn capsules and teas are sold at natural food stores and herb shops.

Motherwort • This herb is a mild sedative and can temporarily reduce blood pressure. It is available at natural food stores and herb shops.

Reishi Mushroom • Compounds found in this delicious mushroom, which is widely used in Asian cooking, can reduce high blood pressure. Reishi mushrooms are available at Asian markets and at better greengrocers.

Immune Weakness

Immunity is a highly complex system involving the interaction of armies of blood cells and proteins that protect the body against microorganisms (such as viruses and bacteria), other foreign substances, and cancer cells. As we age, our immune system becomes less efficient, making us more vulnerable to disease. At one time, it was believed that a weakened immune system was a natural part of the aging process. However, many researchers now suspect that nutritional deficiencies may be a major cause of immune problems in the elderly. Based on these studies, it appears that it may be possible to keep your immune system strong simply by maintaining adequate levels of crucial nutrients and by using appropriate supplements.

EARL'S RX

Beta-carotene • Several studies have shown a higher incidence of various forms of cancer among people with low blood levels of beta-carotene. One explanation is that beta-carotene is an antioxidant, which means that it protects cells against damage by free radicals, which can lead to cancer. However, recent studies suggest that beta-carotene has a specific effect on the immune system. In one important study, twenty-one HIV-positive patients were given very high doses of beta-carotene (180 milligrams, or 300,000 international units) or a placebo. After 4 weeks, the patients on the beta-carotene showed significant increases in several blood factors that fight infection, including T cells, an essential component of the body's defense system. Good sources of beta-carotene include apricots, cantaloupe, broccoli, sweet potatoes, and pumpkin. Beta-carotene is also available in supplement form. Take up to 25,000 international units daily.

Vitamin B$_2$ (Riboflavin) • Studies show that deficiencies in this B vitamin can decrease the number of T cells, which can impair immunity. Good food sources of riboflavin include low-fat milk, yogurt, beef, fortified breads and cereals, and green vegetables. It is also included in B-complex formulas and multivitamins. The recommended daily allowance (RDA) is between 1.3 and 1.7 milligrams. According to *The Surgeon General's Report on Nutrition and Health* (1988), a study of older people reported that more than one-third had low blood levels of riboflavin.

Vitamin B$_6$ (Pyridoxine) • Researchers have found that vitamin B$_6$ depletion in elderly people can result in a depressed immune system. Specifically, B$_6$ deficiency appears to impair the release of interleukin-2 and lymphocyte production, two important parts of the body's defense system. Good food sources include cantaloupe, cabbage, low-fat milk, and blackstrap molasses. B$_6$ is included in many multivitamins and B-complex supplements. The RDA for B$_6$ is 1.6 milligrams for women and 2 milligrams for men. Do not exceed doses over 2000 milligrams. I recommend 100 milligrams daily in a B-complex formula.

Vitamin C (Ascorbic Acid) • Several studies have shown that vitamin C can lessen the duration and severity of the common cold, attesting to its antiviral activity. It also appears to raise blood levels of glutathione, one of the most important antioxidants produced by the body, which also plays a role in immunity. The RDA for vitamin C is 60 milligrams. I recommend 1000 milligrams daily.

Vitamin E (Tocopherol) • A recent study published in *The American Journal of Clinical Nutrition* showed that vitamin E supplements can enhance immune response in healthy people over sixty. In this study, thirty-two healthy adults were given 800 milligrams of vitamin E for 3 days or a placebo. Those taking the vitamin E showed a dramatic boost in immune function but not those taking the placebo. Good food sources of vitamin E include whole grains, vegetable oils, avocados, wheat germ, and sweet potatoes. The RDA is 8 to 10 international units; however, I recommend a supplement of 400 international units daily.

Glutathione • Glutathione is an antioxidant produced naturally in the body. A recent study sponsored by the U.S. Department of Agriculture's Human Nutrition Research Center on Aging at Tufts University has shown that supplements of glutathione can dramatically improve immune function in older people. It not only enhanced the cell's ability to fight infection, but reduced inflammatory substances produced by cells. There is no RDA for glutathione. Take a 50-milligram capsule one or two times daily.

Zinc • According to recent studies, as many as 30 percent of all healthy people over fifty may be deficient in zinc, which could hamper immune function. Researchers at Wayne State University in Detroit gave 3 milligrams of zinc daily to thirteen zinc-deficient men and women. After 6 months, the participants showed signs of improved immune function, notably higher blood levels of thymulin, which is essential for the production of mature T cells. Good food sources include oysters, pumpkin seeds, lamb chops, brewer's yeast, poultry, fortified cereals, low-fat milk, and wheat germ. The RDA for zinc is 12 milligrams for women and 15 milligrams for men. To ensure an adequate amount of zinc, eat zinc-rich foods and take a supplement of 15 to 50 milligrams daily.

Herbal Remedies

Astralagus • Researchers at Texas Medical Center found that a purified extract of astralagus can stimulate T cells in cancer patients with impaired immunity. In addition, other studies have shown that astralagus can increase in the production of interferon, a protein in cells that fights against viruses. Astralagus is available in capsule form at natural food stores.

Echinacea • Several studies have shown that this herb can help the body ward off viral infections. Echinacea has been used to restore normal immune function in cancer patients receiving chemotherapy. It is a traditional Native American treatment for colds and flu. Echinacea is sold as capsules and extract at natural food stores.

Ligusticum (Osha) • Called ligusticum in the Orient and osha in the United States, this herb may boost the body's ability to fight against viruses. It was used by Native Americans to treat viral, fungal, and respiratory infections. Ligusticum or osha capsules and preparations are available at natural food stores.

Shiitake Mushrooms • Lentinen, a compound from shiitake mushrooms, may help activate the immune system and fight against tumor cells. The mushrooms are delicious to eat. Shiitake capsules are available at natural food stores.

Kidney Stones

The kidneys are bean-shaped organs that are located just above the waist. The primary job of the kidneys is to filter waste products from the blood. About 10 percent of all men and 3 percent of all women (usually over forty) will develop kidney stones, a condition that can interfere with normal kidney function and may damage the kidneys.

EARL'S RX

Calcium • Most kidney stones are made of calcium and oxalate, a compound found in many plants. Sources include spinach, tea, wheat bran, chocolate, nuts, and rhubarb. At one time, people with a tendency to develop kidney stones were advised to avoid both calcium and oxalate. However, a recent study suggests that that advice was wrong. In fact, calcium may actually help to prevent kidney stones. Researchers at Harvard School of Public Health studied the diet of more than fifty thousand middle-aged men. Much to their suprise, they found that men who consumed the most calcium were 34 percent less likely to develop kidney stones. The researchers concluded that calcium may have somehow prevented the absorption of oxalate.

Don't Load Up on Oxalates • Although you don't have to avoid foods high in oxalates, you should eat them only in moderation.

Potassium • Based on the same study of fifty thousand men, researchers found that men who ate the most fruits and vegetables had the lowest rate of kidney stones. The researchers speculated that since fruits and vegetables are rich in potassium, this mineral may play a preventive role in the formation of kidney stones.

Increase Your Fluids • Be sure to drink 8 to 10 glasses of filtered water or other nonalcoholic fluids daily. The Harvard

School of Public Health study found that men who drank the most fluids had a 30 percent reduction in risk of developing kidney stones.

Watch the Protein • A high-protein diet has been associated with an increased risk of developing kidney stones.

Macular Degeneration

The macula is a part of the retina that is responsible for central vision—the kind of vision required for activities such as reading fine print, sewing, or driving a car. Macular degeneration occurs when the macula is damaged, leaving a blind spot in the center of the visual field. Macular degeneration is the leading cause of blindness among adults over fifty. Laser surgery may help stabilize vision, but recent studies suggest that vitamins and minerals may help.

EARL'S RX

Pass the Collard Greens • A study performed at the Massachusetts Eye and Ear Infirmary in Boston suggests that a diet rich in spinach and other green leafy vegetables may help to prevent macular degeneration. The researchers compared the diets of 356 men and women (age fifty-five to eighty-five) with advanced macular degeneration to the diets of 520 men and women of the same age group who had some other form of eye disease. The researchers found that the people who ate the most carotenoid-rich food had a 43 percent lower risk of advanced macular degeneration than those eating the least carotenoids. In particular, two carotenoids, lutein and zeaxanthin, both found in spinach and collard greens, appeared to have the most potent protective effect. Interestingly enough, lutein and zeaxanthin form the yellow pigment in the macula of the eye. Although more studies must be done to determine whether these two carotenoids are truly effective against this disease, it makes good sense to include spinach and collard greens in your anti-aging diet.

Antioxidants • A complete antioxidant supplement consisting of alpha- and beta-carotene, vitamins C and E, and selenium, plus green tea and grapeseed extract should be taken daily.

Zinc • Preliminary studies suggest that zinc supplements may help to prevent macular degeneration. Take 15 to 50 milligrams of zinc daily.

Memory Loss

By age sixty, most people will experience some decline in short-term memory and alertness. Ironically, long-term memory may work better than ever; in fact, it may be easier to conjure up the name of a long-lost childhood friend than that of a recent acquaintance. Limited memory loss is not serious, and it is certainly not a symptom of Alzheimer's or senility. Nor is it inevitable that everyone will experience memory loss. In fact, some studies suggest that more than one-quarter of all elderly people perform as well on memory tests as younger people. However, there are several reasons why many older people may find their memory beginning to wane. An older brain may not produce the same quantity and quality of chemicals involved in memory function. The blood supply to the brain could be hampered by atherosclerosis or other circulatory problems. In some cases, medication could be interfering with brain function. Nutritional deficiencies have also been implicated as a factor in memory loss among the elderly. Emotions may also play a role. Some studies have even shown that undue stress can trigger memory loss in the elderly, and boredom and depression may also interfere with brain function. However, diet and supplements may help keep you smart and sharp.

EARL'S RX

Avoid High Blood Pressure • Older people with diastolic pressures over 90 (the bottom number) experience a decline in short-term memory loss, based on a study conducted at the University of Maine. In fact, the longer the person had high blood pressure, the worse the memory loss. However, once the blood pressure is normalized, the memory loss will not deteriorate any further.

Supplements

Vitamin B₁ (Thiamine) • Studies have shown that low levels of this B vitamin can cause subtle changes in brain function among older people that could contribute to memory loss. Good food sources of B_1 include brewer's yeast, unrefined cereal grains, pompano fish, sunflower seeds, ham, and peanuts. The recommended daily allowance for B_1 is 1.0 to 1.5 milligrams for adults. Thiamine is added to most B-complex supplements and multivitamins.

Folic Acid • This B vitamin may prevent memory loss by helping to maintain normal levels of homocysteine, an amino acid found in the body. According to a recent study performed by the Agriculture Research Service of the U.S. Department of Agriculture, researchers found a strong correlation between high blood levels of homocysteine and the loss of memory and the ability to learn that often accompanies depression in the elderly. Other studies have shown that folic acid supplements can normalize homocysteine levels in people with elevated levels. High levels of homocysteine have also been associated with an increased risk of heart disease. Good food sources include dark green leafy vegetables, sunflower seeds, wheat germ, liver, and peanuts. The recommended daily allowance for folic acid is 400 micrograms. Supplements are available at natural food stores.

Choline • The brain uses choline to make acetylcholine, a neurotransmitter that plays a role in memory function. As we age, we begin to produce less acetylcholine, or the acetylcholine that is produced is less efficient, which may be why many older people become forgetful. Some researchers believe that choline supplements can reverse this trend. Good food sources of choline include eggs, soybeans, cabbage, peanuts, and cauliflower. I also recommend phosphatidylcholine, which is actually the active ingredient in lecithin. Take 1200 milligrams daily.

Dimethylaminoethanol • Since the 1950s, this supplement has been dubbed "the smart drug" in deference to its reputed ability to enhance brain function. I recommend 130 milligrams in capsule or liquid form one or two times daily.

Herbal Remedies

Club Moss Tea • Researchers at the Shanghai Institute of Materia Medica recently reported that they had isolated natural compounds in club moss called *huperzine* A and *huperzine* B, which, according to animal tests, helped to improve learning, memory retrieval, and memory retention. (Huperzine A appeared to be the more effective.) Huperzine raised acetylcholine levels by inhibiting acetylcholinesterase, an enzyme that breaks down acetylcholine. Acetylcholine is a chemical found in the brain that is directly involved in memory and awareness. Drink 1 or 2 cups of brewed club moss tea daily. There are several different types of club moss; be sure that the tea is *Huperzia serrata* and not some other species of club moss. (The species of club moss native to the United States has not yet been studied, so there is no way of knowing whether it would be as effective.)

Ginkgo • Animal studies have shown that ginkgo increases the level of dopamine, which improves the body's ability to transmit information. Several human studies have shown that ginkgo can improve mental performance among elderly people who have shown deteriorating mental function. In addition, other studies have shown that ginkgo also improves the blood flow to the brain (and to other vital organs), thus providing the brain with oxygen and nutrients needed to function at peak capacity. Ginkgo is available in most natural food stores and even many drug stores. I recommend a supplement called Ginkgo 24. Take the 60-milligram capsules or tablets two or three times daily.

Sleep Disorders

Sleep disorders, ranging from insomnia to frequent night wakenings, are a major health problem in the United States, especially for people in their middle years and beyond. By age sixty-five, at least half of all Americans experience some form of sleep disorder according to the report *Wake Up America: A National Sleep Alert,* issued by the newly established National Commission on Sleep Disorders Research. Many sleep disorders begin during middle age. In fact, women past forty are at particular risk of developing insomnia, often due to menopausal discomfort.

Sleep disorders not only can severely hamper someone's quality of life, but can have a profoundly negative effect on health. Several studies have shown that lack of sleep can impair memory and make it difficult to concentrate, handle stress, and accomplish daily tasks. In addition, the fatigue caused by inadequate sleep can make you more prone to accidents.

Part of the nation's sleep problem stems from the fact that there are many myths about sleep, and one of the most prevalent is that the older you get, the less sleep you need. In reality, the experts say, if you needed 8 hours of sleep at twenty years of age, you still require the same amount of sleep at forty or even at eighty. And although older people may experience different patterns of sleep than younger ones, such as more frequent night awakenings, very often some of the more severe symptoms, such as chronic insomnia, may be caused by a physical problem such as sleep apnea or an emotional problem such as depression. It could even be something as simple as too much daytime napping or too little physical activity. However, as people age, they may simply accept a bad night's sleep as a way of life. They shouldn't. There are many things that you can do that may help to restore a normal sleep pattern. However, if self-help doesn't work, there are some excellent sleep–wake disorders clinics throughout the United States that have had excellent results. Here are some tips to help you get a better night's sleep.

EARL'S RX

Watch the Stimulants • From early afternoon on, avoiding drinking beverages containing caffeine that could keep you awake at nighttime. Caffeinated beverages include coffee, tea, and many colas and soft drinks. Chocolate also contains caffeine, so avoid eating a candy bar late in the afternoon or evening.

Ditto for cigarettes. I personally think that cigarettes should be avoided all the time; however, if you smoke, keep in mind that nicotine is a powerful stimulant. Try not to smoke too close to bedtime.

Pass on the Nightcap • A shot of booze may lull you to sleep, but it also makes you more prone to nighttime awakenings.

Get Enough Exercise, but Not Too Close to Bedtime • Daily exercise can leave you properly tuckered out at night. However, exercise can have a stimulating effect that can last several hours, so try to finish your exercise routine at least 2 to 3 hours prior to hitting the sack.

Sex • Sex is a natural relaxant that helps soothe the body and promote a good night's sleep. Orgasm triggers the release of chemicals by the brain that are natural pain relievers, which can help relieve any aches and pains that may be keeping you awake.

Avoid Sleeping Pills • Barbiturates can be habit forming and can cause dangerous interactions with other medications. Although it may be tempting to simply pop a pill, in my opinion, the risks far outweigh any advantages. In addition, there are numerous other remedies that work as well without any of the side effects.

Melatonin • Melatonin is a hormone produced by the pineal gland in the brain that helps to regulate sleep–wake cycles. Many scientists have suggested that a reduction in melatonin may be responsible for the disruption in sleep patterns experienced by many older people. The National Institute on Aging is sponsoring studies on the role of melatonin in controlling sleep and wakefulness. Preliminary results have been promising. Recently, researchers at Massachusetts Institute of Technology in Boston have shown that melatonin can quickly induce sleep in volunteers. I use melatonin when I travel to help adjust to different time zones. Take 1 to 2 (up to 5 milligrams) capsules or tablets about 1½ hours before bedtime. Occasional use is preferred. I prefer the sublingual (under the tongue) form. Take ½ hour before sleep; do not drive after taking melatonin.

Herbal Remedies

Chamomile Tea • I always end my day with a cup of chamomile tea. Chamomile has a relaxing effect on the body and is an old-time cure for insomnia. Chamomile tea is widely available at supermarkets and natural food stores. (Chamomile is a member of the daisy family, which also includes ragweed. If you are allergic to any members of the daisy family, avoid this herb.)

Hops • Hops, the flower used to brew beer, can be sprinkled on your pillow for a good night's sleep. Dried hops are available at natural food stores. It really works!

Lemon Balm • This pleasant-tasting herb has long been used to treat nervous tension and insomnia. It is available in tea form at natural food stores. Drink 1 cup daily.

Peppermint • This herb has a soothing effect on the body and may help to promote sleep. In addition, it is excellent for heartburn and stomachache, two conditions that can interfere with sleep. Peppermint tea is sold at supermarkets and natural food stores. Drink 1 cup at night.

Siberian Ginseng • Unlike other forms of ginseng that can cause sleeplessness in some people, Siberian ginseng (*Eleutherococcus senticosus*) is used by Chinese healers to treat insomnia. Siberian ginseng is sold at herb shops and natural food stores as capsules, teas, and extracts. Take 1 capsule up to three times daily or drink 1 or 2 cups of tea daily.

Skullcap • This herb is an old-time remedy for insomnia and muscle tension. It is available at natural food stores and herb shops as capsules and tea. Take 1 capsule up to three times daily, or drink 1 cup of tea daily, preferably toward evening.

Valerian • Herbal healers use valerian to treat insomnia due to anxiety-related problems. Valerian is sold at herb shops and natural food stores in capsule or tea form. Take up to 3 capsules daily, or drink 1 cup of tea daily.

Stroke

A stroke occurs when the brain is deprived of oxygen and nutrients due to the rupture or obstruction of the arteries supplying blood to the brain. Most strokes are caused by blood clots that form in the artery bringing blood to the brain or lodge there from some other point in the body. A minority of strokes are caused when a blood vessel on the surface of the brain ruptures and bleeds or when a defective artery in the brain bursts. The telltale signs of a stroke are sudden weakness or numbness in the face, arm or leg on one side of the body; loss or slurring of speech; difficulty understanding others; sudden and severe dizziness; or headaches. Stroke can result in permanent disability. About 10 percent of all strokes are preceded by transient ischemic attacks, so-called little strokes in which the symptoms disappear within a short time.

Stroke is the third leading cause of death in the United States. The incidence of stroke is directly related to age and sex:

men are three times more likely to suffer strokes than women. Thanks to growing public awareness about symptoms and risk factors, the rate of stroke has sharply declined in the United States. However, more than 500,000 strokes occur each year out which 145,000 are fatal. Sadly, I feel that many of these strokes could be prevented.

EARL'S RX

Watch Your Blood Pressure • High blood pressure is the major risk factor for stroke. (For information on how to control your blood pressure, see p. 209.)

Stop Smoking • If you smoke, you are twice as likely to have a stroke than a nonsmoker.

Maintain Normal Cholesterol • People with coronary artery disease are at an increased risk of having a stroke. High blood cholesterol will increase the odds of developing coronary artery disease.

Watch the Scale • Being overweight can increase your risk of high blood pressure, which in turn will increase your risk of stroke.

Protective Foods

Helpful Veggies • A study of 87,000 female nurses showed that eating lots of carrots and spinach can significantly lower a woman's risk of stroke and presumably a man's, too. Carrots and spinach are rich in antioxidants, including carotenoids, which may help prevent arteries from becoming clogged with cholesterol.

Citrus Fruits • Citrus contains coumarins, natural blood thinners, which may help prevent the formation of clots.

Something Fishy • A landmark Dutch study shows that men who eat more than 20 grams of fish daily (about two-thirds of an ounce) had a lower risk of stroke than those who ate less fish. However, don't go overboard on the fish: a previous study among Eskimos has shown that those who ate the most fatty fish (including mackerel, salmon, sardines, and albacore tuna) had the greatest risk of hemorrhagic strokes. To be on the safe side, stick to two or three fish meals per week.

Garlic • The "stinking rose," as it is sometimes called, contains a compound called *ajoene*, which is a natural blood thinner.

Supplements

Aspirin • Aspirin can prevent the formation of blood clots. Many doctors advise their patients to take a small dose of aspirin (1 baby aspirin) daily or every other day to prevent heart attack and stroke. (No one should take aspirin routinely unless under the supervision of a physician or natural healer.)

Selenium • Studies have shown that people who live in areas with the lowest level of selenium in the soil have the highest rate of stroke. Be sure to eat selenium-rich foods, including garlic, onions, red grapes, broccoli, whole wheat, and chicken. Selenium supplements are available at natural food stores. Selenium is often included in antioxidant formulas. (Doses of over 200 micrograms daily may be toxic.)

Vitamin E (Tocopherol) • Many studies have documented vitamin E's ability to prevent blood clots, which can help prevent stroke. Good food sources include olive oil, whole grains, avocados, sweet potatoes, and oatmeal. Vitamin E is available in supplement form at natural food stores. Take 400 to 800 international units daily.

Herbal Remedies

Ginkgo • This ancient herb improves circulation to the brain and can prevent the formation of blood clots. Ginkgo capsules are available at natural food stores.

Ginger • Ginger prevents "sticky blood," that is, it prevents blood cells from sticking together to form clots. Ginger capsules and teas are available at natural food stores. Ginger is widely used in Asian cuisines.

Ligusticum • Studies have shown that this Chinese herb can help resolve blood clots in patients with transient ischemic attacks and can help improve blood flow to the brain. Ligusticum is available in capsule or liquid form at natural food stores and herb shops.

Taste Loss

As we age, our sense of taste and smell begins to wane. By age sixty, there is usually a noticeable decline in the ability to taste food due to a reduction in the number of taste buds on the tongue. Although the loss of taste is not a medical problem, it can lead to one if it results in a loss of interest in eating, which can lead to malnutrition.

EARL'S RX

Zinc • A daily supplement of 15 to 60 milligrams of zinc gluconate may help to wake up your taste buds.

Check Your Medication • Certain drugs can interfere with the ability to taste food. For example, aspirin can increase sensitivity to bitter flavors, and several other medications such as Biaxin (a form of erythromycin) and tetracycline can cause a lingering aftertaste that can mask the flavor of food. If you're taking medication, check with your physician to see if it could be hindering your taste buds.

Try New Seasonings • Spice up your cuisine—and wake up your taste buds—with a wide variety of herbs and spices. Avoid using too much pepper because it can have a numbing effect on your taste buds.

Variety • Stimulate your taste buds by eating a variety of foods of different textures.

Varicose Veins

A vein is a blood vessel that carries blood back to the heart. (An artery is a blood vessel that carries blood away from the heart.) A series of valves help to push blood through the veins. However, as people age, the valves become less efficient, and skin supporting the veins can become less elastic. As a result, the veins can lose some of their tone, and blood can start to accumulate. After time, the veins can become distended, and varicosities can form. Typically the veins in the legs are most susceptible to becoming varicose, however, other affected sites can include the testes and the esophagus. Varicose veins are not only unsightly, but they can be quite painful.

In some cases, varicose veins are genetic; however, pregnancy, prolonged standing, or even excessive strain of the abdominal region can cause varicosities. Women are four times more likely to develop varicose veins than men, which suggests that hormones may play a role.

In severe cases, varicose veins can be surgically corrected. However, there are some things you can do that may help to prevent this problem.

EARL'S RX

Keep Moving • Although prolonged standing in one spot may cause blood to pool in the legs, exercise can improve circulation. A brisk walk or jog can actually help push the blood through the veins as well as tone up the leg muscles, which in turn help the valves work more efficiently.

Bioflavonoids • Rutin, a bioflavonoid, may help to prevent varicose veins by strengthening capillaries, which are tiny blood vessels. Bioflavonoid supplements are available at natural food stores.

Herbal Remedies

Ginkgo • This ancient herb is used to treat circulatory disorders, including varicose veins. It is rich in bioflavonoids, which may in part explain its beneficial effect on blood flow.

Butcher's Broom • In Europe, this herb is a popular treatment for varicose veins and related disorders. It is available as capsules or a salve that can be placed directly on the affected area.

Gotu Cola • Also known as centella, this herb has been used to treat inflammation and swelling associated with varicose veins. It is available as capsules at natural food stores.

Vitamin E (Tocopherol) • Vitamin E helps to circulate blood to your legs and other extremities. Take 800 to 1200 international units of the dry form in capsules or tablets.

Chapter 4

Just for Women

A s more and more women enter their middle years, I am constantly asked about menopause, breast cancer, and other health-related issues of particular concern to women. In this chapter, I address some of these questions and discuss how women can stay healthy and vigorous for their entire lives.

Sexual Health

Between the ages of forty-five and fifty-five, most women enter into menopause, a time of life marked by profound hormonal changes. During this time, production of estrogen by the ovaries begins to decline, and menstruation becomes erratic and lighter and eventually begins to taper off. Once menstruation stops, the ovaries continue to produce estrogen, but at much smaller quantities. The word *menopause* actually refers to the last menstrual cycle; however, the entire process can take up to several years.

In the United States, the average age for menopause is 51, but heavy smokers can become menopausal up to 10 years earlier, and light smokers up to 3 years earlier.

Menopause affects women differently. Many women experience very few changes and suffer few of the unpleasant symptoms often associated with the "change of life." Others, however, may have a more difficult time adjusting to the sudden fluctuations in hormones.

Millions of American women are taking synthetic hormones (hormone replacement therapy) to help cope with menopausal symptoms. Hormonal therapy is not without risk, which I discuss later in this chapter. There are some tried and true natural alternatives that may ease some of the discomfort of menopause without any of the risk associated with hormone replacement therapy. Here are some common problems that women may experience during menopause and some natural remedies.

Bloating

Hormonal changes in menopause can cause the retention of water, which can result in premenstrual syndrome–type bloating. For some women, the bloating is mild. However, for others, it can be so severe that it is difficult for them to wear anything with a defined waistline.

EARL'S RX

Alfalfa • Also rich in phytoestrogens, the leaves of the alfalfa plant are an excellent diuretic. You can toss fresh alfalfa sprouts in salad, or the dried herb is available as capsules or tea. Take 3 to 6 tablets daily or drink 1 cup of tea daily. **(Caution: Alfalfa can aggravate lupus, an autoimmune disorder. If you have lupus or a lupuslike disease, do not use this herb.)**

Centella • Also known as gotu kola, this herb is a mild diuretic and has also been used to treat depression, another problem that can occur during menopause. Centella is available as capsules. Take 1 capsule up to three times daily.

Dandelion • Dandelion, which is also rich in phytoestrogens, is one of the best natural diuretics. The dried herb is available as capsules and tea. Drink 1 cup of dandelion tea daily or take 1 capsule up to three times daily. Dandelion leaves can also be added to salads. Dandelion is also abundant in potassium, a mineral that is often sapped from the body by synthetic diuretics.

Hawthorn • This herb is known as a cardiotonic because of its positive effects on the cardiovascular system. It is also a mild diuretic. It is available as capsules or tea. Take 1 capsule up to three times daily, or drink 1 to 3 cups of tea.

Other herbal diuretics include wild oregon grape or osha, burdock, nettle, chaparral, celery, and asparagus.

Caution: Many women use licorice root to relieve some of the symptoms of menopause. However, licorice can promote the retention of water and should not be used by women who are prone to bloating or those with high blood pressure.

Dry Mouth

The drop in estrogen can also result in less saliva production, which can create a dry, gritty feeling in the mouth.

EARL'S RX

Water • It seems obvious, but be sure to drink at least 6 to 8 glasses of water daily. Sip water throughout the day to keep your mouth and teeth moist. Chewing sugarless gum or sucking on sugarless candy may help.

Slippery Elm Bark • Cough drops made from this herb may also help to moisturize your mouth.

Synthetic Saliva Sprays • These sprays are sold over the counter and may also offer some relief.

Evening Primrose Oil • Two capsules (500 milligrams each) taken up to three times daily can help this condition.

If all else fails, there are several prescription products available that promote saliva formation that may be helpful. Talk to your physician about which one is right for you.

Fatigue

It is not uncommon for women to complain of excessive fatigue during menopause, which is most often due to hormonal changes. Some women may be awakened at night by hot flashes, others may have difficulty sleeping.

EARL'S RX

Suma • Many herbalists recommend the South American herb suma to treat fatigue. Also known as the South American ginseng, this herb is available at natural food stores. Take 1 to 3 capsules up to twice daily.

Hot Flashes

About half of all American women experience hot flashes during menopause. A *hot flash* is a sudden feeling of intense heat followed by sweating and sometimes chills. For some women, a hot flash can be a temporary nuisance, but for others, it can be debilitating. Hot flashes are caused by hormonal surges by the pituitary, which is trying to stimulate the production of estrogen by the ovaries. Stimulants such as caffeine and alcohol (which is also a depressant) may promote hot flashes.

EARL'S RX

Many women also have found that supplements of vitamin E (400 to 800 international units daily) and vitamin C (1000 milligrams daily) can help prevent hot flashes. In addition, there are other remedies that may help.

Ginseng • Ginseng, an herb that is rich in a plant form of estrogen, has been successfully used by herbalists to treat hot flashes. Ginseng is available in tea and capsule form. Drink 1 or 2 cups of tea daily, or take 1 to 3 capsules. I recommend American or Siberian ginseng; panax ginseng, which is commonly used in the Orient, may be too stimulating for many people and could cause insomnia. In rare cases, ginseng could cause vaginal bleeding. If you experience any irregular bleeding during menopause, alert your physician or natural healer, and be sure to tell her if you're using ginseng. Ginseng should not be used by people with high blood pressure or irregular heartbeats.

Dong Quai • This herb, which is highly prized in the Orient, is known as the female ginseng. It is mildly estrogenic in action and may help relieve hot flashes as well as other menopausal symptoms.

Vitex • This herb, used to regulate hormonal balance—unlike ginseng or dong quai, it is not estrogenic in action—is a very popular menopause aid. Vitex is available as capsules and in "change of life" herbal formulas for women. Take as directed.

Diet • Diet may also help. Interestingly enough, in Japan there is no word for *hot flash*, and its omission from the language reflects the fact that it is a rare symptom among Japanese women. Japanese women eat a diet that is rich in soy foods, such as tofu, tempeh, and soy milk, which are excellent sources of phytoestrogens, plant compounds that behave like estrogen in the body. Researchers speculate that these plant estrogens—although they are much weaker than real hormones—may help relieve some of the symptoms of menopause that are caused by a decline in the production of natural estrogen. Other foods that are rich in phytoestrogens include alfalfa, cherries, barley, apples, rye, potatoes, rice, wheat, yams, and yeast.

Deep Breathing • Deep breathing may also provide relief from hot flashes. In a recent study of thirty-three menopausal women experiencing hot flashes, slow, deep abdominal breathing appeared to cut their rate of hot flashes in half. The researchers suspect that the deep breathing may lower the arousal of the central nervous system, which usually occurs prior to a hot flash. Deep breathing can be used to prevent hot flashes or to try to ward one off if you feel a flash coming on. Simply take slow, relaxed breaths for about 15 minutes. Be sure you're really breathing from your stomach—your abdomen should fill up with air. Do this exercise twice daily.

Mood Swings

Similar to premenstrual syndrome, many women find that they experience mood swings, depression, or irritability during menopause, which are often caused by hormonal swings.

EARL'S RX

The herbs usually given for menopause, including dong quai, vitex, and ginseng, may help promote a feeling of energy and well-being. In addition, try the following remedies:

Vitamin B_6 • This vitamin is commonly used to treat depression or moodiness due to menopause. Take between 50 and 100 milligrams daily in supplement form. In rare cases, doses over 200 milligrams daily could be toxic.

Hops • This herb, which is rich in phytoestrogens, may soothe and help you to relax. It is especially good for women who may be bothered by insomnia. In the old days, people used to sprinkle hops with alcohol, put it in a pillowcase, and sleep on it. Today, hops are available as capsules. Take between 1 and 3 daily.

Ginger • A cup of ginger root tea is a nice pick-me-up.

Vaginal Dryness

The drop in estrogen can cause a thinning in the vaginal lining and a decline in vaginal lubrication. This can result in painful intercourse and makes the vagina more vulnerable to yeast and other infections.

EARL'S RX

Many women have found that vitamin E supplements (400 to 800 international units) can help prevent vaginal dryness. Here are some other things you can try.

Don Quai • Many women rely on dong quai for this and other menopause-related problems. Take 1 capsule up to three times daily.

Wild Yam • This herb is a rich source of plant hormones that may help prevent vaginal dryness. It is available in capsules. Take 1 up to three times daily.

Vaginal Moisturizers • There are many over-the-counter products that can help lubricate the vagina. To avoid potential irritants, be sure to buy one that is unscented.

Kegel Exercises • These simple exercises can help promote circulation to the vaginal lining and maintain vaginal muscle tone. Squeeze your vaginal muscles—it should feel as if you're trying to stop urinating midstream—hold in your muscles tightly for about 10 seconds, and then release. Repeat this exercise for up to 10 minutes twice daily.

Yeast and Urinary Tract Infections

The thinning of the vaginal and urethral lining make women more prone to yeast and urinary tract infections.

EARL'S RX

Lactobacillus acidophilus • This so-called friendly bacteria found in yogurt may help prevent yeast infections. If yeast infections are a problem, eat 2 cartons of yogurt daily (which is also a terrific way to get calcium) or take 2 acidophilus capsules ½ hour before or after meals three times daily.

Cranberry Capsules • These may help to prevent urinary tract infections. Take 2 capsules up to three times daily or drink 2 glasses of unsweetened cranberry juice daily.

Uva ursi • This herb is commonly used to treat urinary tract infections in women and men. Take 1 capsule up to three times daily to relieve symptoms.

Breast Cancer

Breast cancer is the second leading cause of cancer deaths among American women; lung cancer has the dubious distinction of being the number one cancer killer. In 1994, about 200,000 were diagnosed with this disease, and 46,000 died from it. Breast cancer is a very serious problem; however, the oft-quoted figure that one out of nine women will get breast cancer is somewhat misleading. The risk of developing breast cancer dramatically increases with age. Therefore, a twenty-year-old woman has a significantly lower risk of getting breast cancer than a forty-year-old, and a forty-year-old woman has a significantly lower risk of getting breast cancer than a sixty-year-old, and so on.

The incidence and mortality rate of breast cancer is much higher in western Europe and the United States than it is in Asia or Africa. For example, American women are four times more likely to die from breast cancer than are Japanese women. Yet, when Japanese women migrate to the United States, within one or two generations, their mortality rate from breast cancer is equal to that of the native population. Researchers speculate that breast cancer may be caused by environmental factors such as diet or exposure to cancer-causing chemicals.

Genetics may also play a role in breast cancer, but it appears to be a small one. Only about 6 percent of all cases of breast cancer are believed to be linked to heredity, which means that more than 90 percent of all cases of breast cancer occur in women who have no previous family history of this disease.

Why is the rate of breast cancer so high in the Western world? Is there anything a woman can do to reduce her risk? Although we don't have all the answers, there is some compelling evidence that diet and lifestyle may help prevent breast cancer.

THE LOWDOWN ON FAT

One obvious difference between the United States and countries such as Asia and Africa is diet in general and fat in particular. Our diet contains nearly two to three times the amount of fat as is eaten in less-developed countries. In particular, Westerners eat much more saturated fat, notably from dairy and animal products. In the human body, hormones are stored in fatty tissue. The female hormone estrogen has been shown to trigger the growth of estrogen-sensitive tumors in the breast and other parts of the body. (More than half of all breast tumors are estrogen sensitive.) Therefore, it's possible that a diet high in fat could result in more fat stores in the body and higher levels of hormones. In addition, in menopausal women, hormones produced by the adrenal gland are converted into estrogen by fat cells, which could explain why obesity is a risk factor for breast cancer among menopausal women.

Fat is also the storage site for many potentially dangerous carcinogens that we get from food and other sources that could also spur the growth of tumors.

Epidemiological studies, that is, studies of large populations, have shown a definite link between the consumption of fat and a higher rate of breast cancer among women. For example, in the United States, Seventh-Day Adventists, many of whom are vegetarians and consume less fat than the general population, have up to a 75 percent reduced risk of dying of breast cancer. In addition, animal studies have shown a direct correlation between a high-fat diet and the growth of breast tumors. However, human studies have been more ambiguous. In fact, a major study of nurses published in *The Journal of the National Cancer Institute* showed that there was little difference in the fat intake of women who developed breast cancer and those who did not. Critics of the study, however, contend that all the women in the study were eating too much fat—on average, over 30 percent of their daily calories—and that if women would reduce their fat intake to under 20 percent of daily calories, there would be a significant decrease in the incidence of breast cancer.

Another study revealed that out of a group of women with estrogen-sensitive tumors who have had mastectomies, those who ate a high-fat diet prior to surgery were more likely to suffer a relapse of breast cancer than those who ate leaner fare.

More research is needed to determine if a very low fat diet can significantly reduce the rate of breast cancer, and as of this writing, there are some studies exploring that question. However, given the fact that a high-fat diet has also been implicated in heart disease, diabetes, obesity, and a slew of other medical problems, I think it makes good sense to keep your daily fat intake to between 20 and 25 percent of daily calories.

ENVIRONMENTAL ESTROGENS

For more than a decade, scientists have known that certain chemicals and pollutants in the environment can disrupt normal biological processes in humans and animals. When these compounds are broken down in the body, they mimic the action of hormones such as estrogen. And similar to naturally produced hormones, these "chemical" hormones can trigger the growth of breast tumors and other cancers. Dichlordiphenyltrichloroethane (DDT), which was once widely used as an insecticide but was banned in 1972, is still causing trouble. DDT is broken down in the body to an even stronger compound, dichlordiphenylethylene. There is no evidence that DDT causes cancer, but studies have shown that women with breast cancer have significantly higher rates of dichlordiphenylethylene in breast tissue than women who are cancer free. DDT is not the only culprit. Other compounds that can have similar estrogenic effect in the body include ingredients in plastics, laundry detergents, and some other legal pesticides.

It's very hard to completely avoid many of these chemicals because they are ubiquitous in our environment. However, my philosophy is that you can try to avoid as much personal contact with these chemicals as possible. For example, to reduce pesticide exposure, eat only organically grown fruits and vegetables. Organic produce is available at natural food stores and many supermarkets. Although it costs a bit more, I think it's worth the difference. It's also wise to avoid saturating your lawn or garden with chemicals. Fortunately, there are many natural toxin-free lawn and garden products on the market that can do the job just as well. Check your local plant nursery, natural food store, or botanical gardens for information on environmentally friendly gardening techniques.

Try to avoid potential household toxins. Although we really don't know which, if any, of these products can raise the risk of developing breast cancer, I think it makes good sense to take some precautions. Avoid using aerosol sprays of all types; buy products that come in a pump bottle. Wear gloves when you're using cleansers to prevent skin contact. And avoid unnecessary products such as room deodorizers.

HORMONE REPLACEMENT THERAPY

Millions of women take a daily dose of synthetic hormones—estrogen and progesterone—to help alleviate some of the unpleasant symptoms and side effects of menopause. Studies show that in addition to preventing symptoms such as hot flashes, hormone replacement therapy can help prevent heart disease and osteoporosis. However, there is a downside to pumping your body full of synthetic hormones: women on hormones significantly increase their risk of breast cancer and uterine cancer. In fact, women age sixty to sixty-six on hormone replacement therapy have an 87 percent increased risk of breast cancer. At a recent meeting of the American Association for the Advancement of Science, Dr. Graham Colditz of Harvard Medical School asked an important question: should breast cancer be the price we pay for reduced risk of heart disease and bone fractures? His answer was no, and so is mine.

In the previous section on menopause, I detailed many natural and safe alternatives to hormone replacement therapy. I strongly advise women to think twice before doing anything that will increase their odds of becoming another breast cancer statistic.

ALCOHOL

There is a great deal of confusion about the possible link between alcohol and breast cancer. Some studies have shown that women who drink alcohol increase their odds of developing breast cancer. In fact, in a recent Spanish study of more than 760 women with breast cancer, there was evidence that even moderate drinking (1 or 2 drinks daily) increased the risk of developing breast cancer by 50 percent. However, other studies have not found any connection between drinking and breast cancer.

However, a recent study did find a connection between alcohol intake and estrogen levels. In a 1993 issue of *The Journal of the National Cancer Institute*, researchers reported that women who drank about 1 ounce of pure alcohol daily (roughly two average drinks) showed higher blood and urine levels of estrogen than when they abstained. Because estrogen can promote cellular growth in breast and reproductive tissue, this is a cause of concern, particularly for women who are at risk of getting breast cancer. Given this information, I feel that women with family histories of breast cancer should probably drink only very occasionally if at all. It's also advisable for women who are already taking synthetic estrogen in the form of birth control pills or hormone replacement therapy to think twice about ingesting a substance that will boost their estrogen levels even higher.

FIBER

Several studies have shown that a high-fiber diet reduces the risk of developing breast cancer. There are several reasons why fiber may offer some protection. For one thing, foods that are high in fiber, such as fruits, vegetables, and grains, tend to be low in fat. For another, these foods are also rich in phytochemicals that may help prevent the initiation and spread of many different forms of cancer. Finally, there is some evidence that a particular form of fiber—wheat bran—may help to lower the level of estrogen. In a study conducted by the National Health Foundation, premenopausal women were given 30 grams daily of either wheat bran, corn bran, or oat bran. After 2 months, only the women on the wheat bran showed a significant reduction in serum estrone and estradiol, two potent estrogens that are believed to stimulate the growth of breast tumors. Researchers believe that the estrogen binds with wheat fiber and is eliminated in the feces.

CANCER FIGHTERS

There are several other foods and supplements that are believed to have a protective effect against breast cancer.

Carotene • One study performed at the Department of Social and Preventive Medicine at the State University of New York at Buffalo, compared the diets of 439 postmenopausal women with breast cancer to postmenopausal women who were cancer free. The researchers found that the risk of breast cancer was highest among women with the lowest intake of carotene in their food. Although the study appeared to deal with only beta-carotene, it's important to note that foods that are rich in beta-carotene are also often good sources of alpha-carotene, lutein, and other carotenoids. Apricots, bok choy, pumpkin, carrots, and cantaloupe are excellent sources of carotenes.

Vitamin C • Several studies have linked a low intake of vitamin C with an increased risk of breast cancer.

Genistein • Found only in soy products, this compound has been shown to block the growth of breast cancer cells in test tube studies. Many people believe that the low rate of mortality from breast cancer among Japanese women is due to their high consumption of soy products. Tofu, soy milk, and soy protein is a good source of genistein.

Legumes • Legumes such as soybeans, lentils, and kidney beans are also believed to protect against breast cancer. Dried beans contain many anticancer compounds including phytic acid and protease inhibitors. They are also low in fat.

Lignans • Found in abundance in flaxseed and to a lesser extent in rye, lignans are hormonelike compounds that compete with the body's own estrogen for estrogen receptor sites on cells. By doing so, lignans deactivate potent estrogens that may trigger the growth of breast tumors.

Limonene • Found in the peel of citrus fruits, this compound has been shown to inhibit the growth of carcinogen-induced mammary tumors in rats and prevent new tumors from forming.

Omega-3 Fatty Acids • Found primarily in fatty fish, such as salmon, mackerel, and albacore tuna, studies have shown that omega-3 fatty acids can inhibit the growth of mammary tumors.

Quercetin • Studies show that this bioflavonoid can inhibit the growth of human tumor cells containing binding sites for type II estrogen, which may be responsible for some forms of breast cancer. Quercetin is abundant in red and yellow onions and shallots.

Sulforaphane • Found in broccoli and other cruciferous vegetables, sulforaphane promotes the production of anticancer enzymes in the body. In one study, rats were pretreated with either a high dose or a low dose of a synthetic form of sulforaphane and then given a carcinogen known to induce mammary tumors. Another group of rats were just given injections of the carcinogen. More than two-thirds of the group that did not receive the sulforaphane developed breast cancer, as opposed to 35 percent of the low-dose sulforaphane-treated group. Out of the high-dose sulforaphane group, only 26 percent developed cancer.

PERSONAL MAINTENANCE

There are no guarantees with cancer: you can do all the "right things," eat the right foods, take the right vitamins, and for some unknown reason still develop breast cancer. However, the earlier the stage in which breast cancer is diagnosed, the better the prognosis. Therefore, women should be vigilant about examining their breasts for lumps or signs of abnormalities at least once a month. If you don't know how, the American Cancer Society has some excellent pamphlets that can show you what to do.

Most women should have a baseline mammogram by age forty, and some should have one earlier depending on family medical history. By age fifty, women should have an annual mammogram. Be sure to get your mammogram at a facility that is accredited by the American College of Radiology.

Lung Cancer

Lung cancer actually kills more women annually than breast cancer. Although some cases of lung cancer may be genetic or even related to diet, in many cases, lung cancer is a self-inflicted disease, and cigarettes are the weapon of choice. Since women have started smoking, there has been a steady rise in the incidence and mortality rate from lung cancer. In fact, since the 1980s, mortality rates from lung cancer among women have increased 3 percent annually. Women smokers have more than five times the risk of developing lung cancer than nonsmokers.

I know it's not easy to quit. Cigarettes contain highly addictive substances that are designed to keep you coming back for more. However, keep in mind that it's not just your lungs that are in jeopardy. There is nothing that will age a woman faster than a cigarette. Women who smoke enter into menopause on average 2 years earlier than nonsmokers. They also are more prone to develop osteoporosis. In addition, they develop more wrinkles on their skin and look on average about 5 years older than nonsmokers.

Some forms of lung cancer are not related to smoking, and in these cases, dietary fat may be a major culprit. In a study conducted by the National Cancer Institute, researchers surveyed 1450 nonsmokers ages thirty to eighty-four. Out of this group, 429 had been diagnosed with lung cancer between 1986 and 1991. Based on this study, the 20 percent of the women who ate the highest amount of saturated fat had six times the risk of developing lung cancer than the 20 percent of the women who ate the least amount of saturated fat. Researchers aren't sure if fat per se is the "smoking gun" or whether fat was present in some other food, such as cooked red meat, which also contains potential carcinogens such as heterocyclic amines.

One interesting note: in this study, the women who ate the most beans (legumes) and peas had a 40 percent lower risk of lung cancer than those eating the least!

Osteoporosis

Osteoporosis is caused by the thinning or wearing away of bone, which increases the susceptibility to breaks and fractures. Areas that are particularly vulnerable include the vertebrae, hips, and forearms. About four out of five of the 25 million Americans with osteoporosis are women, and the majority are menopausal. Small-boned white and Asian women are at greatest risk of developing this disease. Hispanic and African-American women are at the lowest risk.

Nearly 40 percent of all postmenopausal American women will suffer vertebral fractures, and in severe cases, some will develop a rounded back or dowager's hump. Osteoporosis is not merely an aesthetic problem: it can be very serious, even fatal. About 15 percent of all white women over fifty will fracture a hip sometime in their lifetime. About 20 percent of women hospitalized for hip fractures will develop medical complications such as pneumonia or blood clots that will result in their deaths. Osteoporosis is a growing problem. By 2030, the U.S. National Institutes of Health estimates that the rate of hip fractures will reach 400,000 annually, up from 300,000 in 1994.

Osteoporosis can also cause tooth loss due to bone deterioration in the jaw.

Losing bone is a natural part of the aging process and happens in both men and women. However, osteoporosis is the rapid loss of bone. During childhood and early adulthood, new bone is constantly being produced. Bone consists of several minerals including a large amount of calcium and phosphorus salts and smaller amounts of magnesium, zinc, iodine, fluoride, and other trace elements. By around age thirty, people develop their peak bone mass, that is, the production of new bone cells begins to slow down. In fact, after thirty-five, people begin to lose roughly 1 percent of their bone mass annually. After menopause, however, women begin to lose about 2 to 4 percent of their bone mass each year for up to a decade until it begins to level off. The rapid loss after menopause is attributed to a decline in estrogen, which is essential for calcium absorption. In fact, many menopausal women are given hormone replacement therapy (also known as estrogen replacement therapy, which has been shown to stem the rapid bone loss associated with menopause). However, hormone replacement therapy is a short-term solution. If a woman goes off hormones, as many do after 5 years, the rate of bone loss begins to accelerate. In addition, many women cannot take hormones in the first place.

Women who cannot or will not take hormones or who don't stay on hormones for their entire postmenopausal lives are not doomed to get osteoporosis. Osteoporosis is not an inevitable part of aging: with proper planning and intervention, it can be prevented. There are many things that a woman can do throughout her lifetime to keep her bones healthy and strong.

CALCIUM AND VITAMIN D

Several studies have underscored the need to get adequate amounts of calcium and vitamin D. Vitamin D is essential to help the body utilize calcium and phosphorus. Some forms of osteoporosis may be caused by a genetic inability to utilize vitamin D correctly, which adversely affects the body's ability to absorb calcium. In fact, researchers have recently isolated the gene that may be responsible for the malfunction in vitamin D absorption.

The recommended daily allowance (RDA) for vitamin D is 400 international units. (Vitamin D can be toxic at levels over 1000 international units daily. Do not exceed the RDA unless under a physician's supervision.)

The RDA for calcium is 800 milligrams for children up to 10, 1200 milligrams up to age 24, and 1000 milligrams for adults. Most adults consume roughly half the recommended amount. However, the National Osteoporosis Foundation recommends that postmenopausal women not taking estrogen replacement therapy should consume 1500 milligrams of calcium daily. There is even some evidence that 800 milligrams daily may be low for girls. In one study, adolescent girls consuming about

1600 milligrams of calcium were shown to develop significantly stronger bone mass than girls consuming less calcium. The researchers noted that the high-calcium consumers were not excreting excess calcium in their urine, which suggested that during adolescence when these girls were building their peak bone mass, the body was retaining the extra calcium. Although most experts do not recommend that parents give children more than 800 milligrams, it is imperative that children get the full RDA.

Even after peak bone mass is formed, calcium is needed to retain the bone you have. Many researchers believe that maintaining calcium levels during the thirties, forties, and fifties will help boost calcium stores, which women can draw upon in later years. There is also some evidence that increasing calcium levels during menopause may make a real difference. In one 1992 French study of 3270 women over age sixty-five, researchers gave half the group supplements of 1200 milligrams of calcium and 800 international units of vitamin D. The other half received a placebo. After about a year and a half, the vitamin-supplemented group had 43 prevent fewer hip fractures than the unsupplemented group. In addition, hip bone density increased in the supplemented group by 2.7 percent and actually decreased by 4.6 percent in the unsupplemented group.

Good food sources of calcium include low-fat or no-fat dairy products (one nonfat plain yogurt contains about 400 milligrams). However, many low-fat cheeses contain phosphate, which may interfere with the body's ability to absorb calcium; therefore, these foods are not a good calcium source. Other good food sources of calcium include tofu processed with calcium sulfate (434 milligrams per 4 ounces), sardines with bones (324 milligrams per 3 ounces), calcium-fortified orange juice (220 milligrams per 6-ounce serving), and broccoli (90 milligrams per 4 ounces, cooked). Calcium can also be obtained through supplements. There are many different types of calcium supplements; I recommend calcium citrate because it is the best absorbed. Supplements that contain calcium citrate contain less calcium per dose (about 200 milligrams) than some other forms of calcium, which means that you need to take more pills.

Calcium citrate should be taken on an empty stomach.

Beware of supplements made from bone meal, oyster shells, or dolomite; recent studies show that they may contain unsafe levels of lead.

Vitamin D is present in fortified daily products (1 cup of milk provides 100 international units) and fatty fish oils. Sunshine is also an excellent source of vitamin D, because ultraviolet rays stimulate certain skin oils to produce vitamin D. However, sunscreens and sunblocks may filter out the rays necessary to produce vitamin D. Therefore, it's important to expose your skin to sun without protective lotion once or twice a day for about 10 minutes. Limit your sun exposure to the very early morning (before 10 A.M.) or late afternoon (after 3 P.M.) when the sun is not at its strongest.

For many women, it may be necessary to supplement vitamin D during the winter when bone loss occurs at a faster pace than during the warmer months. In fact, according to a recent study, a supplement of 400 international units of vitamin D during the winter can reduce bone loss. Talk to your physician or natural healer about increasing your intake of vitamin D during the winter.

EXERCISE

A regular program of weight-bearing exercise may help strengthen bones. In fact, the lack of physical activity in our modern-day lives may be one of the major reasons why osteoporosis is on the rise. Studies show that human bones are actually getting weaker. For example, during the restoration of an old church in London, scientists compared the bone density of eighty-seven women buried in a church crypt from 1729 to 1852 to the bone density of postmenopausal women living today who were roughly the same age. The scientists discovered that the dead women had denser bones and appeared to have lost bone at a much slower rate than the contemporary women. The scientists were puzzled by the result but attributed the denser bones of the deceased women to the fact that they were probably much more physically active than women today. Without modern conveniences such as washing machines and cars, these women performed more physically demanding tasks. Studies have shown that weight-bearing exercise, such as walking, running, or jogging, can not only help build bone but will increase muscle mass, which can protect against fractures by absorbing the shock of a fall. (Swimming and cycling are not weight-bearing exercises.)

Combining calcium supplements with exercise may offer added protection. Researchers at Tufts University studied the effect of calcium and exercise on the bone density of thirty-six postmenopausal women. One group of women was given a high-calcium drink daily containing 831 milligrams of calcium, whereas the other group was given a low-calcium (41 milligrams) placebo. Each woman was told to include 800 milligrams of calcium in her diet. In addition, women were either assigned to participate in an exercise group (a 50-minute walk four times per week) or were told to refrain from any recreational activities. After 1 year, the researchers found that the women consuming the most calcium had a 2 percent increase in the femoral neck bone mineral density, whereas the placebo group had a 1.1 percent decrease. In addition, the exercise group showed a 0.5 percent increase in the bone mineral density of the spine, whereas the sedentary group experienced a 7 percent decline. This and other similar studies show that diet and lifestyle can make a significant difference in reducing the risk of osteoporosis.

MEDICATION

A drug called salmon calcitonin is one of two Food and Drug Administration–approved treatments for postmenopausal bone loss (estrogen is the other). Calcitonin is a hormone produced by the thyroid gland and is found in humans and many animals. Calcitonin helps to regulate the amount of calcium in the blood and by doing so indirectly affects the amount of calcium in the bone. Studies show that calcitonin can actually stop bone loss and is also used to relieve pain from fractures. Calcitonin may also stimulate new bone formation. Calcitonin is safe, but there may be some unpleasant side effects such as nausea. The real downside to calcitonin is that it must be delivered daily by injection; however, many people can do this on their own with little difficulty. In Europe, a nasal spray form of this drug is available, which may be sold in the United States within a few years. If you have osteoporosis and are not taking hormone replacement therapy, talk to your physician about using calcitonin.

OTHER BONE BUILDERS

There are other foods and supplements that may help to preserve bone.

Boron • Researchers at the U.S. Department of Agriculture found that a supplement of 3 milligrams of boron daily could double serum estrogen levels in women, which may help to prevent osteoporosis. Estrogen helps to retain adequate amounts of calcium and magnesium, which are needed to build strong bones. Good food sources of boron include dried fruit and grapes.

Soy Foods • Even though Japanese women are small boned, they suffer about half the number of hip injuries as American women. The fact that they may be more active physically may be one reason why they have fewer injuries. For example, Japanese women typically sit on the floor, and the action of getting up and down several times daily may help to develop their hip bones. However, their diet, which is rich in soy foods, may be another reason why they have stronger bones. Researchers at the University of North Carolina investigated the effect of genistein, which is found in soybeans, on the bone mass of rats who had their ovaries removed to eliminate their natural source of estrogen. Genistein is rich in plant estrogens, compounds that mimic the action of natural estrogen in the body. The study determined that genistein was able to prevent bone loss in rats almost as well as a synthetic form of estrogen. Although more studies need to be done, soy appears to be a bone-sparing food that American women should include in their diet. (Tofu made with calcium sulfate is a particularly good choice: it is abundant in both calcium and genistein.)

WATCH THESE BONE BREAKERS

Caffeine can hamper calcium absorption. In a 4-year study performed at the University of California of nearly one thousand postmenopausal women, researchers found that those who drank 2 cups of coffee per day or more suffered a significant drop in bone density. However, those who drank at least 1 cup of milk per day seemed to be protected from coffee's bone-breaking effect.

Smokers have a higher rate of osteporosis than nonsmokers. Yet another reason to kick the habit!

Alcohol can hamper the absorption of calcium, which will cause bones to become thin and brittle. Excessive drinking also makes you more prone to falling, which can result in a break or fracture.

Chapter 5

Just for Men

Men typically die younger than women. I don't believe that men are the "weaker sex," rather, men are more stoic about their health—they often ignore important symptoms and deal with health problems only when they absolutely have to (or when their wives force them to!). However, a new generation of men is taking a greater interest in health and fitness, and I believe this change in attitude may add years to the average man's lifespan. Here's some important information that every man should know about.

Sexual Health

Good health and great sex go hand in hand at any age, but it is particularly true for men once they reach middle age. As men approach the second half of life, hormonal shifts and other changes can alter sexual response. Hormone levels that control sexual arousal may dip. For example, many men showed a marked drop in testosterone production beginning around in their late forties. In Europe, this period is called *viropause*, and there are some similarities to the female menopause. Similar to female menopause, some men may experience minor symptoms resulting from hormonal fluctuations. Although men remain fertile, they may find that it takes longer to get an erection and they may have difficulty maintaining one at times. However, none of these factors should significantly impair a man's ability to enjoy sex.

There is no intrinsic reason why a man can't enjoy a vigorous sex life for his entire life. However, many men do not. According to the Massachusetts Male Aging Study, a recent groundbreaking study of men between the ages of forty and seventy, about half of the 1290 participants experienced some form of impotency. The researchers defined impotency as "the persistent inability to attain and maintain an erection adequate to permit satisfactory sexual performance." Most of the men experienced minimal or moderate forms of impotency. The risk of severe or total impotency increased threefold with age: 5.1 percent of all forty-year-olds complained of complete impotency versus 15 percent of all seventy-year-olds. But the researchers were quick to point out that in most cases, a persistent sexual problem was a sign of an underlying physical problem. In fact, 39 percent of the heart disease patients and 15 percent of the high blood pressure patients were completely impotent compared with less than 10 percent of the entire group. (In these situations, the impotency is often not due to the disease, but to the medication that is used to treat it, as I will discuss later.) Disregard for one's body also seemed to be a major culprit in promoting impotency. For example, for heart patients, smoking appeared to be the kiss of death for sex: those who lit up were three times more likely to be impotent than those who did not.

The study also revealed that the men least likely to complain of impotency were those with high levels of high-density lipoprotein, or "good" cholesterol. In addition, contrary to popular opinion, blood testosterone levels were not related to male potency. But another hormone was right on target: blood levels of dehydroepiandrosterone (DHEA), which is produced by the adrenals, were a good indicator of impotency. (For more information on DHEA, see p. 171.) In fact, men with the highest levels of DHEA were the least likely to be impotent. This doesn't necessarily mean that DHEA promotes sexuality; its effect on a man's sex life may simply be due to the fact that men with high DHEA levels are less likely to develop heart disease.

Many of the physical problems that can destroy a man's sex life are easily avoidable or can be successfully treated. The following section reviews some of the major causes of male impotency and ways to cope with them.

Poor Circulation

In order to maintain an erection, blood must flow freely to the penis. However, if the arteries delivering blood to the genitals become narrowed or clogged due to atherosclerosis, the blood supply will be impaired. This could explain why so many heart patients complain of impotency. Diabetics, hypertensives, and heavy smokers are also at great risk of damage to their vascular system, which could result in a poor blood flow to their genitals. Impotency is often the first sign of a circulatory problem in men.

EARL'S RX

A low-fat diet (with less than 20 percent of daily calories in the form of fat) is your best defense against clogged arteries. If you smoke, stop. Each and every cigarette you smoke inflicts slow damage to your vascular system, which will eventually result in circulatory problems. In addition, if you smoke, your partner may also light up. Smoking can impair a woman's vaginal lubrication, which will make having sex even more difficult.

If you are diabetic, be especially vigilant about maintaining normal blood sugar levels. There is evidence that high blood sugar can cause nerve damage that can contribute to impotency. The combination of cigarette smoking and diabetes appears to be particularly dangerous.

To improve blood flow throughout the body including to the sex organs, take a vitamin E supplement of 400 international units twice daily, morning and evening. (Do not take vitamin E if you are using a blood thinner.) In addition, the Chinese herb *Ginko biloba* has also been shown to improve circulation to the extremities. *Ginko biloba* is available in capsule form at natural food stores.

Alcohol

Although a drink or two may help you "loosen up," contrary to popular belief, alcohol actually inhibits erection and ejaculation in men. Heavy drinkers may damage their liver, thus impairing the production of sex hormones. In addition, chronic alcoholics may permanently damage nerves within their penis that are essential to maintain an erection.

Earl's RX • If sex is on your agenda, hold off on the alcohol until you're done. If you're a heavy drinker, talk to your physician about getting help to stop.

Drugs

Prescription and over-the-counter drugs can cause many sexual problems in men. Some medications, including those used to treat high blood pressure, depression, anxiety and even allergies, can sap sexual desire or cause impotency or difficulty with ejaculation. For example, some men on beta-blockers used to treat hypertension may experience what I call the "beta-blocker blues," a palpable loss in libido. In addition, men on antidepressant drugs such as amitriptyline hydrochloride (Elavil) may suffer a loss of libido or find that they have difficulty with ejaculation. Finally, some men may respond to certain medications with excessive fatigue: although they may be physically capable to have sex, they may feel too dragged out.

EARL'S RX

I don't want to panic men who may be on prescription drugs: these kinds of adverse reactions to drugs are relatively rare, affecting between 1 and 2 percent of users. However, if a man is experiencing impotency or other sexual problems and he is taking medication, he should check with his physician to determine if the medication could be causing the problem. Oftentimes, simply switching to another medication will solve the problem.

Caution: If you are on medication for heart disease, high blood pressure, or any other serious problem, do not discontinue your medication without first checking with your physician.

If you are hypertensive and suspect that your blood pressure medication is bringing you down, it may be possible to reduce your dose simply by adopting certain changes in your diet and lifestyle. Be sure to work closely with your physician or natural healer so that he or she can monitor your results.

If you're taking medication for a heart problem, keep in mind that fear may be hampering your sexual performance, not your medication. Many heart patients mistakenly believe that they cannot withstand the physical stress of sex. In most cases, this is simply not true. In fact, one recent study concluded that for most heart patients, having sex was no more dangerous than getting out of bed in the morning! Talk to your physician or natural healer about your fears.

Fatigue or Loss of Desire

If you simply can't summon up the energy or the interest to have sex, you need to reexamine your lifestyle. Are you getting enough sleep? Are you getting enough exercise? Are you eating a healthful diet? Are you knocking yourself out at night with a nightcap? Could you be suffering from a vitamin deficiency? Excessive fatigue could be a sign of depression or an underlying physical problem, so if you are constantly exhausted, you should consult with your physician or natural healer. However, very often, it's a sign of poor nutrition and poor health habits.

EARL'S RX

Vitamin A • Vitamin A helps produce sex hormones that are essential for sexual functioning. Eat foods rich in beta-carotene, which is converted into vitamin A as the body needs it. Take 10,000 to 15,000 international units of beta-carot daily.

Vitamin B$_6$ • B$_6$ boosts the levels of hormone that regulates testosterone. Good food sources include brewer's yeast, wheat germ, cantaloupe, cabbage, and blackstrap molasses. A good multivitamin will contain B$_6$.

Manganese • This mineral helps produce two chemicals in the brain that heighten sexual arousal: dopamine and acetylcholine. Good food sources of manganese include nuts, whole grain breads, cereals, legumes, beets, and green leafy vegetables.

Zinc • Zinc is essential for the production of testosterone. (As I discuss later, it also helps to keep the prostate gland healthy.) Men should take between 15 and 50 milligrams of zinc daily.

Octacosanol • This natural food supplement, which is rich in wheat, wheat germ, and vegetable oils, is reputed to increase stamina and sexual performance in some men. Octacosanol is sold in capsule form in natural food stores.

Yohimbe • This herb is the only Food and Drug Administration–approved aphrodesiac on the market for men. The drug yohimbine is available by prescription only and has been shown to restore sexual potency in some men. The herb yohimbe, a much weaker version of the drug, is available in natural food stores and is included in many so-called male potency formulas. I recommend 500-milligram capsules up to two or three times daily.

Following my simple suggestions may help some men. However, any man who has a chronic problem with impotency should see his physician or natural healer. Fortunately, there are numerous medical treatments available for impotency including surgical penile implants. Don't suffer in silence, talk to your physician.

Prostate Problems

The prostate is a small walnut-sized gland located between the bladder and the penis, above the rectum. The prostate gland produces semen, the fluid that carries sperm. During childhood, the prostate is tiny; however, once puberty kicks in and testosterone levels rise, the prostate gland grows to adult size. The prostate gland remains stable until around age forty-five, at which time it often experiences a second growth spurt. By age sixty, most men have an enlarged prostate gland, a condition that is called *benign prostate hypertrophy* (BPH). As its name implies, in most cases, BPH is harmless, although it can be quite annoying. If the prostate gland becomes very swollen, it can push against the urethra and interfere with urination. In fact, in about 10 percent of all men, the first sign of BPH is urinary retention. Other symptoms include difficulty or straining during urination and frequent urination, especially at night. In severe cases, urine can gather in the bladder until it eventually backs up into the kidneys, causing kidney damage. About 10 percent of men with BPH will require corrective surgery; in fact, prostate surgery is the most common surgery performed on people over sixty-four.

Earl's RX • Some men may find that certain foods, such as caffeinated beverages, alcoholic drinks, and hot, spicy food, may aggravate their condition. Obviously, if you find certain foods or drinks to be irritating, your best bet is to avoid them. However, many men with BPH try to cope with their problem by drastically reducing their intake of liquids. This is not a good idea and could actually add to their woes by triggering a urinary tract infection. If you have BPH, consult with your physician or natural healer. Most men can be treated successfully with medication or with any number of herbal remedies that may relieve some of their discomfort.

In 1992, the Food and Drug Administration approved a new drug, finasteride, marketed as Proscar, for BPH. Proscar works by blocking the conversion of testosterone into a more potent form of the hormone that is believed to trigger prostate growth. Proscar works well for many men but is expensive and can cost up to one thousand dollars annually. A small number of men on Proscar experience impotency and decreased libido among other side effects. In addition, Proscar should not be used by people with liver problems.

Natural food stores are also filled with prostate remedies, some of which work well for many men. Natural remedies tend to work better in the early stages of BPH. The advantage of using a natural remedy is that it is inexpensive and can be purchased without a prescription. The downside of herbal remedies is that they are much weaker than the prescription drugs and may not work for everybody. On the positive side, however, they do not cause any known side effects. For many men, herbal remedies will do the trick. However, if the herbal remedy doesn't help, they can always switch to a stronger medication. Following are some popular remedies that may help men with BPH.

Saw Palmetto • Many herbal formulas for BPH contain extract from the berries of the saw palmetto tree. Native Americans ate saw palmetto berries as part of their diet. Natural healers have long prescribed these berries for urinary problems.

Several studies have shown that saw palmetto can increase

the flow of urine and reduce nighttime urination in men with BPH. In Europe, where most of the research on saw palmetto was conducted, this herb is an accepted treatment for BPH.

Some studies show that saw palmetto berry extract may work by preventing the conversion of testosterone to its more potent form, dihydrotestosterone. Compounds in the saw palmetto berry may block dihydrotestosterone's ability to bind to receptor sites on prostate cells, thus preventing the cells from growing. Take 1 to 3 capsules (540 milligrams) daily.

Pygeum • The bark of the pygeum plant has been used for prostate problems since the eighteenth century and is included in many modern herbal formulas. Pygeum contains phytosterols, compounds that have anti-inflammatory activity. Phytosterols block the production of prostaglandins, compounds that are involved in the inflammatory process. In addition, pygeum is a diuretic, which can help promote urination.

Pumpkin or Squash Seeds • A species of pumpkin or squash seeds grown in the Near East *(Cucurbita pepo)* is included in many herbal prostate formulas. *Curcurbita pepo* contain many beneficial phytochemicals including beta-sistosterol, an anti-inflammatory, and cucurbitacin, which may help facilitate urination by relaxing the sphincter (that regulates the flow of urine and increasing the tone of bladder muscles. Pumpkin seeds are also an excellent source of vitamin E and zinc.

Pumpkin seed oil is sold in natural food stores in capsule form.

Stinging Nettle • This herb is a a diuretic and anti-inflammatory. It is often in conjunction with the herbs discussed above to treat prostate problems.

Couch Grass • This mild diuretic is often included in many herbal combinations for BPH.

Zinc • Zinc plays a major role in the male reproductive system. There are heavy concentrations of zinc in the prostate gland. Zinc stimulates the production of testosterone, the male hormone that aids in men's capability for erection and ejaculation. A zinc deficiency may contribute to infertility. Zinc may also help to prevent BPH. Therefore, I advise men to take 15 to 50 milligrams of zinc daily and to eat foods rich in zinc, which include pumpkin seeds, oysters, cashews, nonfat dry milk, brown mustard, pork loin, round steak, and brewer's yeast.

CANCER OF THE PROSTATE

Cancer of the prostate is the second most common form of cancer in American men. (Skin cancer is number one.) In 1994, some 200,000 American men will be diagnosed with this disease.

Responsible for 35,000 deaths annually, prostate cancer is the second leading cause of cancer deaths among men, surpassed only by lung cancer. In the United States, the lifetime risk of getting prostate cancer is one out of eleven for white males and one out of nine for African-American men. The death rate from prostate cancer is steadily creeping upward by about 2 to 3 percent annually. African-American men are three times as likely to die from prostate cancer as white men, probably due to late diagnosis.

In most cases, if caught early, prostate cancer can be successfully treated by surgery or radiation therapy. In many older man (over sixty), however, the tumors are so slow growing that they may not need treatment at all. In these cases, the physician may recommend a policy of "watchful waiting" to see how the cancer progresses.

Because of the risk of prostate cancer, men over forty should have an annual physical examination that includes a digital rectal exam. In this exam, the physician inserts a lubricated finger into the rectum to palpate for any prostate irregularities or early rectal cancers. However, the digital rectal exam may not detect small tumors. That is why the American Cancer Society recommends that men over fifty also have an annual prostate-specific antigen (PSA) blood test. PSA is a protein produced by the prostate. High levels of PSA may be a sign of tumor growth.

All men should be aware of the warning signs and symptoms of prostate cancer. According to American Institute for

Cancer Research, men should report any of the following symptoms to their physicians.

- Any changes in urinary habits.
- Blood in the urine.
- Painful urination.
- Continuing pain in the lower back, pelvis, or upper thighs.

Keep in mind that having one or more of these symptoms does not mean that you have cancer. It could also be a sign of a urinary tract infection or another problem and should not be ignored. Even if it does turn out to be prostate cancer, the earlier the diagnosis, the better the prognosis.

In the United States, prostate cancer is relatively common, but not so in Asia or Africa. In fact, Japanese men have the lowest rate of mortality from prostate cancer in the world. Black men in Nigeria have a lower rate of prostate cancer than African-American men in the United States. Researchers suspect that diet and other environmental factors may contribute to the risk of dying from prostate cancer.

In one major study conducted at Harvard Medical School of 48,000 men, researchers found that diet may play a major role in determining who lives or dies from prostate cancer. In this study, researchers compared the diets of the 417 men out of the group who had been diagnosed with prostate cancer to those of the men who did not get this disease. The researchers found that diet did not appear to increase the odds of developing prostate cancer. However, among the men who developed this disease, a diet high in fat appeared to be a major risk factor in whether or not the disease emerged to a more advanced state. Animal fat in particular appeared to have a lethal effect on prostate cancer. Specifically, men who ate the highest amounts of red meat, butter, and chicken with skin fared the worst. However, eating skinless chicken, vegetable fat, or dairy products other than butter did not seem to have any adverse affect. From this information, researchers concluded that a particular form of fatty acid—alpha-linolenic acid found in animal sources—may be responsible for triggering tumor growth. It's interesting to note that other studies have shown that Seventh-Day Adventist men who follow a vegetarian diet have a much lower rate of prostate cancer than the national average. And even though Japanese men in Japan have an extremely low rate of mortality from prostate cancer, when they migrate to the United States—and presumably begin eating the typical American diet—their risk dramatically increases.

Another reason why Japanese men in Japan may be protected against prostate cancer is the fact that their diet is rich in soy foods such as tofu and soy milk. In my book *Earl Mindell's Soy Miracle*, I reviewed numerous studies that showed that many of the compounds in soy have potent anticancer properties. Soy is rich in phytoestrogens, hormonelike compounds that may deactivate the more potent hormones that can trigger tumor growth. One compound in particular, genistein, has been shown in test tube studies to inhibit the growth of prostate tumor cells. Genistein is now being tested on men in the United States who are in the early stages of prostate cancer to see if it can slow down the progress of the disease. Interestingly, autopsies of Japanese men reveal that their rate of prostate cancer is as high as that of American men. Most of them have small tumors in their prostates when they die; however, these tumors are not detected because they are so slow growing, they never develop into clinical disease. Studies will show whether or not genistein is the secret weapon against prostate cancer. Given the epidemic of prostate cancer in the United States, I recommend that men try to eat at least one serving (2 to 3 ounces) of tofu or soy food daily. I start my morning with a tofu shake. There are also powdered soy protein products on the market that offer a day's supply of genistein.

Other Male Concerns

HAIR TODAY . . .

Some men manage to keep a thick head of hair throughout their entire lives, but starting around middle age or even younger, most men experience hair loss that could eventually lead to balding. Healthy, young men lose an average of about 100 hairs daily, which are usually replaced by new growth. As men age, however, hair may tend to thin out and, in some cases, result in balding.

About two-thirds of all men have male pattern baldness, which is a genetic condition passed down by either parent. However, even if one of your parents is bald, it doesn't mean that your fate is sealed. The gene can skip a generation. However, the reverse is also true: even if your parents have thick, lustrous manes, you could still inherit the gene for baldness.

Male pattern baldness usually begins gradually, starting with a loss of hair at the front of the scalp at either side of the hairline or on the crown, the circular area on top. Hair loss can start as early as the teenage years, but more often than not, it begins during middle age.

Why so many otherwise healthy men lose their hair as they age is still very much a mystery. Some researchers believe that testosterone, the male hormone, may thwart hair growth by shrinking the hair follicle. Others believe that the hair follicle becomes clogged with sebum, a substance produced by the skin, which prevents nutrients from reaching the hair follicle, thus thwarting growth.

In some cases, hair loss may be caused by an underlying physical problem. For example, an underactive or an overactive thyroid can create a hormonal imbalance that can accelerate hair loss, but once the problem is corrected, the hair grows back. Cancer patients may suffer temporary hair loss after radiation or chemotherapy treatments. Sometimes rapid hair loss is a sign of an autoimmune disease called *alopecia areata*, which results in patchy bald spots on the scalp. However, hair loss due to alopecia is usually temporary in adults. In extremely rare cases, a severe vitamin deficiency may be the underlying cause.

For thousands of years, men have sought a cure for baldness. To this date, there is no tried and true cure for this problem. However, there are some treatments that may help some people.

A handful of men have had success with the drug minoxidil, marketed under the name Rogaine. Since 1979, minoxidil has been given orally to treat hypertension in patients in whom other drugs have not worked. Sold under the name Loniten, minoxidil had some scary side effects, including rapid heart rate, fainting, breathing difficulties, and the accumulation of fluid around the heart. Minoxidil had one other interesting side effect: physicians prescribing minoxidil noticed that it promoted hair growth on the scalp and other parts of the body including the hands, cheeks, and nose. Because minoxidil is a strong drug that could produce many dangerous side effects, it could not be prescribed orally to treat a cosmetic problem like baldness. However, researchers at Upjohn Company, the makers of minoxidil, devised a minoxidil–alcohol solution that could be applied directly to the scalp, thus eliminating many of the side effects associated with the oral form. In 1989, the Food and Drug Administration approved the external use of minoxidil, or Rogaine, to treat baldness.

No one is sure why minoxidil may help to grow hair. Some experts speculate that it works by stimulating the flow of blood to the scalp, which may stimulate the hair follicle. Others feel that minoxidil may counteract the balding gene in a cell, instructing hair follicle cells to grow although they may have been programmed to shut down.

How well does minoxidil work? Based on several studies, it appears that only a small number of men will experience noticeable hair growth. For many men, however, minoxidil will produce a disappointing fuzz or no results at all. For maximum result, minoxidil treatments should begin at the first sign of baldness. The solution must be rubbed into the scalp twice daily. If the minoxidil is discontinued, hair loss will resume.

Minoxidil is expensive; treatment can cost up to $100 dollars monthly. The usual dose is a 2 percent minoxidil solution; however, if the low dose fails, some physicians may prescribe up to a 5 percent solution.

Studies show that external minoxidil does not appear to produce any of the dire side effects of oral minoxidil. However, some physicians are still reluctant to give the drug to people with an existing heart condition. A small number of men who have used minoxidil complained of itching on the exposed areas, which was probably due to the alcohol.

There is one natural alternative to minoxidil that may or may not work for you, but it's a lot cheaper and you don't need a prescription. Jojoba (pronounced ho-ho-ba) oil, which is made from a desert plant, can also improve the blood flow to the scalp. After shampooing, massage a few drops of oil into your scalp and keep it on overnight. Be sure to avoid contact with your eyes, and if any irritation occurs, discontinue use. Shampoo out in the morning.

Diet and nutrition play a major role in how you feel, and how you feel is reflected in how you look. Although a healthy lifestyle may not prevent hair loss, it can help keep your remaining hair in peak condition. For a healthy, shining mane, be sure to eat foods rich in B vitamins. Brewer's yeast, wheat germ oil, raw and roasted nuts, and whole grain foods are packed with B vitamins.

As the baby boom generation grows up—the generation that turned long hair into a political statement—there is likely to be a frantic search for a cure for baldness. For example, researchers are investigating the possible use of Proscar, a drug designed to treat enlarged prostate glands, to treat baldness. Proscar works by keeping testosterone levels under control, which may help to reduce hair loss. One Canadian company is even experimenting with a machine that zaps the scalp with low-level electricity, which supposedly stems hair loss by stimulating the hair follicles.

When it comes to balding, men will try practically anything. Native Americans used to rub chili peppers on their scalp to stimulate hair growth. This is not as crazy as it sounds: similar to minoxidil, chili peppers stimulate blood flow to the hair follicles, allowing nutrients to flow freely. I don't recommend this treatment because chili peppers can be very irritating to the skin and eyes; however, it's interesting to note that the so-called hot new treatments of today are not really that hot or new.

SAVE YOUR SKIN

Skin cancer is the most common cancer to afflict men. Men are more likely to die from melanoma, the potentially lethal form of this disease, than are women. Not so coincidentally, men spend nearly twice as much time in the sun as do women and are four times less likely to use a sunscreen.

I can't stress this enough: if you are exposed to the sun, you must use a sunscreen of at least 15 sun protection factor (SPF) at all times. Make sure that the sunscreen offers broad-spectrum protection, which means that it filters out both ultraviolet A and B rays.

Keep in mind that sunscreens are not a panacea. Recent studies show that although sunscreens can help prevent basal cell and squamous skin cancers, both of which are highly treatable if caught early, they do not protect against the more serious melanoma. Try to avoid sun exposure during the "burning rays" of 10 A.M. to 2 P.M. However, if you spend a great deal of time outdoors, for example, if you work outside during the summer months, I recommend wearing sun-protective clothing. Dark clothing with a heavy weave offers the best protection; however, it's likely that it will also keep you uncomfortably warm. A summer-weight T-shirt offers protection equal to an SPF of 5 to 7 and only a 2 SPF when it is wet. Fortunately, there are some new lines of lightweight clothes that are specifically designed to offer additional sun protection. There are at least three manufacturers that claim their outerwear offers an SPF of 30. Look for sun-protective clothing at your local sporting goods store.

Don't forget to wear a hat. It not only offers additional protection for your face, but shields your scalp from the cancer-causing rays.

Men who feel that summer is just not summer without a tan should investigate using a self-tanning cream. In the past, these creams fell into disrepute because they turned the skin a sallow yellow color. However, the new creams produce a better result and in my opinion are a much safer alternative to a suntan.

SAVE YOUR BLADDER

It's conventional wisdom that people should drink between 8 and 10 glasses of water daily, and I know many active men who drink even more. Water helps prevent constipation, keeps the skin moist, and helps maintain the correct balance of fluids in the body. A recent study, however, showed that men who drink 14 or more cups of fluid daily of any kind—including coffee or fruit juice—face a two to four times greater risk of developing bladder cancer than men who drink around 7 cups. Further investigation showed that tap water—whether it was consumed in pure form or in fruit juice or brewed coffee—appeared to be the culprit. Researchers speculate that chlorine in municipal water systems may promote cancer. My advice: keep drinking water, especially in the hot summer months, but switch to bottled water or install a home filtering system.

Testosterone

At one time, researchers believed that the male hormone testosterone was the primary reason why men fell prey to heart disease at younger ages and had a shorter life span than women. However, recent studies suggest that testosterone may have been getting a bad rap. For example, one important study performed at Saint Luke's–Roosevelt Hospital Center in New York showed that contrary to previous assumptions, men with lower levels of testosterone were more likely to get heart disease than men with higher levels. In addition, men with higher testosterone levels had higher levels of high-density lipoproteins, or "good" cholesterol.

Testosterone levels tend to decline with age, and some researchers speculate that providing supplemental testosterone to men with low levels may help to ward off some age-related ailments. For example, studies have shown that testosterone supplements in older men may help to prevent osteoporosis, maintain muscle strength, control depression, increase sex drive, and even help to boost brain function. In fact, some researchers speculate that in the not too distant future, many older men may routinely take testosterone supplements much the same way that many menopausal women take estrogen replacement therapy. There is one downside to testosterone: similar to estrogen, it can stimulate the growth of hormone-sensitive tumors and may contribute to prostate cancer. My advice: as good as testosterone therapy may sound, proceed with caution.

Chapter 6

Getting Physical: The Power of Exercise

Since early times, men and women have been desperately searching for a fountain of youth—a magical pill or potion that could reverse the aging process. Fortunately, the search is over and the fountain of youth may be as close as your local gym. Study after study confirms the fact that exercise may be the one true way to turn back the clock. I'm not talking about becoming a marathon runner or an Olympic athlete; a moderate and consistent exercise program is all it takes to live longer, live stronger, and live better.

As we age, there are many physical changes that affect strength and appearance. For most people, by age forty-five, there is a noticeable decline in muscle mass and an increase in body fat. In fact, the typical sedentary adult loses up to 7 pounds of lean body mass per decade. There is also a decrease in bone density; bones get thinner and more prone to fracture.

Aerobic ability declines, which means that you may find yourself huffing and puffing more after exertion. There is also a loss of flexibility; you may feel stiffer and less supple. However, aging does not have to be a physical downward spiral. Many of these changes can be postponed, minimized, and even reversed by physical activity. In fact, experts say that a fit fifty- or sixty-year-old can actually be in better shape than a flabby thirty-year-old! In addition, exercise may help prevent many of the diseases that can cut life short.

Exercise: The Best Preventive Medicine

LONGEVITY

A recent study of ten thousand Harvard graduates ages forty-five to eighty-four showed that those who participated in moderately vigorous activities (such as tennis, swimming, jogging, and brisk walking) had up to a 29 percent lower death rate than the sedentary men. In fact, exercisers on average lived 10 months longer than those who did not exercise. Interestingly, even men who began exercising late in life (after age sixty-five) lived up to 6 months longer than couch potatoes.

In another study performed at the Institute for Aerobics Research and the Cooper Clinic in Dallas, researchers followed thirteen thousand men and women for an average of 8 years to determine whether there was any correlation between fitness levels and longevity. Based on the results of an exercise treadmill test, the group was divided into five levels ranging from the least fit to the most fit. The women in the least fit group had the highest mortality rate. However, women in the second lowest fitness group had nearly half the death rate of the least fit. Based on these findings, the researchers concluded that something as easy as taking a brisk walk daily could add years to your life.

HEART DISEASE

In the same study of ten thousand men in the previous section, those who exercised had a 41 percent reduced risk of heart disease than sedentary men. This is not surprising, considering that other studies have shown that regular exercise can decrease your total cholesterol, increase the "good" high-density lipoproteins, improve respiratory function, and lower your blood pressure. In another study conducted at the Laboratory of Cardiovascular Science at the Gerontology Research Center in Baltimore, researchers found that physical activity may retard the increased stiffness in arteries that often accompany aging. The scientists studied fourteen middle-aged long-distance runners who ran about 30 miles a week. They found that the runners had a greater capacity to dilate their coronary arteries than sedentary men of the same age, thus markedly increasing the blood flow to their heart. Researchers aren't sure how much activity is required to keep arteries from stiffening, but they do know that being sedentary is a sure way to speed up the process.

STROKE

In a 22-year follow-up of more then 5300 Japanese-Americans in the famous Honolulu Heart study, researchers found a strong association between a sedentary lifestyle and an increased risk of stroke. In inactive and partially inactive men between ages fifty-five and sixty-eight, there was a fourfold risk of hemorrhagic stroke (bleeding in the brain) and threefold risk of subarachnoid stroke (bleeding between the brain and the skull) when compared to active men.

Exercise also appears to protect women against stroke. Researchers at the University of Washington in Seattle investigated exercise intensity and early signs of cardiovascular disease in about twelve hundred women. The scientists found that the women who exercised the least were most likely to show signs of thickening of the inner and middle layers of the carotid arteries in the neck, which could increase the risk of stroke.

CANCER

Exercise appears to offer a protective effect against different forms of cancer. Many animal studies have shown that exercise can inhibit tumor growth. There's some evidence that increased physical activity may zap cancer cells in humans as well. For example, a recent study showed that men with sedentary jobs were 1.6 times more likely to develop colon cancer than those with more active jobs. Researchers speculate that physical activity causes an increased motility of the gastrointestinal tract and more frequent bowel movements, which limits exposure to potential carcinogens in stool.

There is also a link between exercise and lower rates of breast cancer. In a major study performed at the Harvard School of Public Health, researchers tracked the exercise habits of 5400 women graduates ages twenty-one to eighty. Based on the study, the more athletic the woman, the lower her risk of developing breast cancer. Other studies have shown that exercise can reduce estrogen levels; some forms of estrogen can trigger the growth of tumor cells.

IMMUNITY

Exercise may add some zip to your immune system. Exercise heats up the body much the same way a fever raises your temperature. When the body is warm, it triggers the production of pyrogen, a protein that is part of interleukin, a type of white blood cell that enhances immune function. Other studies suggest that exercise may reverse the drop in immune function that normally occurs with aging. Researchers at Appalachian State University in Boone, North Carolina, found that very fit women over seventy had immune systems that functioned as well as women half their age!

A word of caution: long-distance running may actually dampen your immune system. Studies show that runners are more prone to colds, flu, and upper respiratory ailments after participating in a marathon. Researchers suspect that overexertion may have a weakening effect on the body. Moderation is the key!

PREVENTING FRAILTY

Researchers are learning that exercise can keep you active and mobile at any age. According to a groundbreaking study conducted at the Hebrew Rehabilitation Program for the Aged in Boston, a carefully planned strength training program for the elderly can counteract muscle weakness typical of very old people. The study found an average 113 percent increase in muscle strength among the participants, which in many cases meant the difference between eating alone in their rooms and being able to walk to the dining room. On average, the exercisers experienced a 12 percent increase in walking speed and a 28 percent increase in stair climbing power. An added bonus: the people who exercised began to take part in more recreational and educational activities offered at the home, thus enriching their lives in other ways. Researchers suspect that if more older people participated in strength training programs, many could avoid the kinds of falls and injuries that force them into nursing homes in the first place. Other studies have shown that men as old as ninety showed a significant improvement in muscle strength after a mere 8 weeks of exercise.

MENTAL FITNESS

Flexing your muscles may strengthen your brain power. Researchers have documented that older people who do regular aerobic exercise perform significantly better on cognitive tests than their sedentary colleagues. One explanation could be that exercise improves blood flow to the brain.

MENTAL WELL-BEING

Exercise makes you happier. Physical activity increases the release of beta-endorphins, chemicals produced by the brain that are natural painkillers. Exercise also lowers your adrenaline level, which can reduce feelings of stress and anxiety.

OSTEOPOROSIS

Weight-bearing exercise can help slow down the loss of bone mass, which is particularly problematic in postmenopausal women. Researchers suspect that regular exercise could help women retain up to 5 percent of their bone mass—women on average lose up to 35 percent of their bone mass in the years following menopause. Beginning an exercise program before menopause will lay down a foundation of bigger and stronger bones.

Getting Started

TAKE THIRTY

Half of all Americans are sedentary, that is, they barely get any physical activity at all. Many people say that they'd like to exercise, but with their busy schedules, they simply can't find a chunk of time during the day to work out. In addition, many people were put off by exercise gurus who insisted that fitness could only be achieved by following a complicated and rigorous program. The good news is, they were wrong. According to the President's Council on Physical Fitness, all it takes to achieve a reasonable level of fitness is to exercise moderately for at least 30 minutes daily. It doesn't have to be in one continuous session—you can do a little bit of exercise throughout the day as long as it adds up to a total of 30 minutes.

Design an exercise program that works best for you. For example, it can be as simple as taking a brisk walk twice daily for fifteen minutes (or three walks for 10 minutes each). Or you can work out on an exercise bike for fifteen minutes in the morning before work and take a fifteen-minute walk after work. Have a back-up plan for bad weather. An indoor jogging track or shopping mall is a great place to walk or run on nasty days. Don't worry if you miss a day; as long as you exercise on most days, you're ahead of the game. Jogging, running, tennis, and swimming are also good choices. Or try something more exotic, such as fencing or martial arts. Many older people are discovering that studying tai chi can help build strength, grace, endurance, and confidence.

STRETCHING

In addition to the 30-minute activity program, I recommend that everyone do some simple stretching exercises at least three times a week for 15 minutes at a time to help maintain flexibility. It's not difficult: simply get down on the floor and gently stretch and flex every joint and bone in your body. Start with your toes and work your way up. Breathe slowly and deeply into the stretch, and stop if you feel any pain or discomfort. Even better, take a stretch and tone class at a health club or local Y. Even if you just attend one stretch class weekly, you can do the exercises at home on your own. There are also some excellent exercise videos on the market that include stretching and strengthening. One of my favorites is *Body Electric* with Margaret Richard. The videotape is fun and easy to follow. In addition, her show is featured on many public television stations and is a great way to start the day. *The Wellness Encyclopedia,* written by the editors of *The University of California, Berkeley, Wellness Letter,* includes a terrific section on exercise that provides specific information on working out at home.

STRENGTH TRAINING

Several studies have shown that strength training with weight can preserve flexibility, muscle, and bone in people well into their nineties. I don't recommend buying a set of weights and working out on your own; the chance of injury is too great. However, I do recommend learning how to use weights properly at a health club or Y. Hire a personal trainer to work with you for a few sessions so that you can learn how to use weights safely. In some cases, the facility may even provide new members with a few free sessions with a trainer. Be sure the trainer is accredited by the American College of Sports Medicine; there are many people out there claiming to be qualified exercise trainers but who have few qualifications.

HELPFUL TIPS

Find an exercise partner. It's more fun to have company, and you're less likely to slack off if another person is counting on you. It's also safer not to run or walk alone, but even with a partner, avoid walking in deserted areas. Be sure to wear reflective gear at night, especially if you're walking on a road that is used by cars.

If you have a heart condition or any other medical problem, check with your physician before beginning an exercise program.

Are You Getting Enough of What You Need?

Exercise places new demands on your body. Be sure that you are getting enough of these important vitamins and minerals.

CHROMIUM

Chromium helps to burn fat and regulate blood sugar. Combined with exercise, chromium can help build muscle. Many Americans are deficient in chromium. Good food sources include spices such as cinnamon, grape juice, brewer's yeast, broccoli, mushrooms, whole wheat, apples, and peanuts. Chromium supplements are sold in natural food stores. Take a 200-microgram capsule or tablet up to three times daily.

VITAMIN B₂ (Riboflavin)

This B vitamin helps the body release energy from food. Researchers at Cornell University found that the need for riboflavin increases with activity. Many studies show that older people do not get enough of this vitamin. Good food sources include low-fat milk, yogurt, lean beef, fortified breads and cereals, and green vegetables. Riboflavin is included in many multivitamins and B supplements. Take 50 to 100 milligrams daily.

VITAMIN E (TOCOPHEROL)

Although exercise offers many benefits, several studies have shown that vigorous exercise increases oxygen consumption, which may promote the formation of free radicals. Free radicals are unstable molecules that can destroy cells. However, antioxidants, particularly vitamin E, may help prevent this damage. In fact, studies also show that vitamin E supplements can help prevent muscle soreness that often occurs after a workout. It's difficult to get enough vitamin E from food alone. Therefore, I recommend taking 800 international units daily in the form of D-alpha-tocopheryl succinate (dry form).

POTASSIUM

Sweating can sap the body of important minerals including sodium, which most of us have enough to spare, and potassium, which can be replaced by eating potassium-rich foods. Fruits such as bananas, orange juice, and prunes are excellent sources of potassium. So are baked white potatoes and plain yogurt.

WATER

While you are exercising, take a few sips of water every 10 minutes or so. Don't forget to drink at least 2 glasses of water after working out.

ZINC

Increased physical activity can lead to a loss of zinc in sweat and urine. Zinc-rich foods include pumpkin seeds, oysters, low-fat milk, brewer's yeast, and lamb chops. Zinc is included in many multivitamins. Take 15 to 50 milligrams daily.

Chapter 7

Looking Good and Staying That Way

Nothing can make you look older than wrinkled, dried-out skin. But skin is not just for decoration: in reality, it is the largest organ system in the body and one of the most hardworking. Skin performs many critical tasks: it helps regulate body temperature; it enables the body to retain fluids; and it's the immune system's first line of defense against viruses, bacteria, and other foreign objects.

As we age, skin undergoes normal wear and tear. Fine lines and wrinkles may develop, which are caused primarily by a breakdown in *collagen*, the protein that is responsible for the support and elasticity of the skin. Gravity begins to pull the skin down, which can cause it to loosen and become flabby. The body produces less *sebum*, an oil that forms a protective coating on the skin, which can result in patches of dry, itchy skin. Cell regeneration slows down, which can leave the skin looking drab and tired. Perhaps the worst assault to skin is caused by exposure to ultraviolet (UV) light from sunlight, which can damage skin cells and cause premature aging and skin cancer.

Until recently, we believed that there was little that could be done to prevent the skin from showing signs of age. However, we now know that a combination of factors, including lifestyle, diet, supplements, and skin care products, can help skin maintain a youthful appearance and, more importantly, keep skin cancer free.

Getting Back to the Basics

Healthy habits are reflected in healthy, glowing skin. Before investing a lot of money in fancy products, try these simple things first.

BEAUTY IS FROM THE INSIDE OUT

Skin is made of cells, and cells need the proper nutrients to thrive. A careful diet including an abundance of fruits, vegetables, and fiber can help keep your body working well and your skin in top form. In addition, studies have shown that a low-fat diet (no more than 20 percent of your calories from fat) can reduce the risk of developing precancerous skin lesions (actinic keratoses) that can lead to nonmelanoma skin cancer, the most common cancer among white Americans. Vitamins and other supplements can also help. In particular, I recommend the following.

Earl's Rx for Beautiful Skin

RNA/DNA, 100 milligrams each daily
Superoxide dismutase and wild yams, 300 milligrams each
daily
Cysteine, 500 milligrams
Vitamin C, 1500 milligrams
Biotin, 100 micrograms
Beta-carotene, 25,000 international units
Water, 6 to 8 glasses daily of filtered or bottled water

GET YOUR BEAUTY SLEEP

During sleep, our bodies secrete human growth hormone and
other skin growth factors that may stimulate the production of
collagen and the production of new skin cells. A chronic lack of
sleep may take its toll on your complexion.

SMOKING

According to a report in *The New England Journal of Medicine*,
smokers are more likely to appear at least 5 years older than
nonsmokers. Smoking is associated with an acceleration in facial wrinkling, perhaps because smokers are constantly squinting their eyes to avoid smoke from their own cigarettes.

WATER

If you don't get enough fluids, your body will sap fluid out of
body cells, which can leave them dehydrated. Dehydrated skin
cells are more likely to have a dried-up, wrinkled appearance.
The antidote is easy: drink 8 to 10 glasses of water daily. (A glass
or two of juice is fine, but remember that many juices are laden
with calories.)

EXERCISE

Moderate exercise can relieve tension, and tension can add years to your face. A stressed-out twenty-year-old with "worry lines" on her forehead can look older than a relaxed and fit forty-year-old.

MAINTAIN NORMAL WEIGHT

Constant weight loss and gain can rob skin of its flexibility, resulting in sagging skin.

BE GENTLE

Don't tug or pull at your face. Cleanse gently with a cotton ball or soft washcloth, and pat dry. Loofas and grainy cleansers are often too rough for many people and should be used rarely on skin if at all. People with dry skin should avoid abrasive cleansers altogether.

Sun Protection

As far as your skin is concerned, UV light is public enemy number one. According to the American Cancer Society, about 700,000 new cases of skin cancer will be diagnosed this year, most of them due to sun exposure. Although most cases of skin cancer are not serious, more than 32,000 people develop malignant melanoma, which is potentially fatal. The bad news is, it appears that sunscreens and blocks do not protect against melanoma. Sun exposure can also accelerate the aging process. In fact, dermatologists blame as much as 80 percent of the skin damage associated with aging on exposure to the sun. As dangerous as the sun may be, I'm not suggesting that people spend their days indoors. However, be sure to follow these guidelines.

NO TAN IS A GOOD TAN

Until recently, the prevailing philosophy had been that if you gradually increased your exposure so that you didn't burn and wore a good sunscreen, it was possible to tan safely. We now know that there is no such thing as a good tan. Tanning is the body's response to injury; therefore, it should be avoided.

AVOID PEAK EXPOSURE

Do as my friend the dermatologist does: during the summer, he runs for shelter during the hours of 10 A.M. and 2 P.M., when the sun is the strongest. Confine your outdoor activities to early morning or late afternoon.

CHECK YOUR MEDICATION

Some medication, such as tetracycline, Retin-A, and even some diuretics, can increase sensitivity to the sun. If you're taking any medication, be sure to check with your physician before spending time outdoors.

WEAR SUNSCREEN

Wear a sunscreen with a sun protection factor (SPF) of 15 daily. Sunscreens come as high as 50 SPF, but many people may find these stronger screens to be irritating and not more effective than an SPF of 29. The SPF means that you can stay out in the sun that many times longer with the sunscreen on without burning than without it. Even if you use a waterproof sunscreen, always reapply sunscreen after swimming or sweating or at least every 2 hours. Apply your sunscreen at least a half an hour before going out in the sun; it takes time to soak into the skin.

A good sunscreen should protect against both UVA and UVB rays. UVB rays can cause wrinkling and damage to your skin. UVA, once believed to be safe, have also been shown to cause significant skin damage. For the best protection, use a broad-spectrum sunscreen that can reflect UV rays as well as absorb them. For example, some sunscreens contain titanium dioxide, a chemical that reflects UV light off the skin and is often used in so-called chemical-free sunscreens. (In reality, no sunscreen is chemical free; rather, the active ingredient sits on top of the skin and does not get absorbed.)

Many people may be allergic to some of the ingredients used in sunscreens. For example, PABA (*para*-aminobenzoic acid), a common ingredient, may trigger a rash of irritation in some people. In some cases, reflective sunscreen may be less irritating because it doesn't interact with the skin. Many brands of sunscreen now claim to be hypoallergenic, which means they are less prone to cause a rash or irritation. Others claim to be noncomedogenic or nonacnegenic, which means that they are less likely to clog pores. No matter what the manufacturer may claim, if you are sensitive to skin products in general, be sure to try a sunscreen on a small area of skin before using it all over your body. If the area remains irritation free for 24 hours, the product is probably safe for you. If in doubt, check with your physician.

If your skin dries out in the sun, be sure to use a sunscreen with a moisturizer. Aloe vera is still my favorite, and it is included in many sunscreens. It is also good to help heal skin after too much sun exposure.

Of course, it's critical to wear sunscreen in the summer when you're outdoors more; however, many dermatologists advise their patients to use sunscreens all year long, at least on their faces. In fact, many brands of makeup now include SPF protection. Using a foundation with a sunscreen is an easy way to make sure that your face is protected daily.

BRONZERS

There are several products on the market that can help you tan without ever stepping foot in the sun. These products contain dihydroxyacetone, which I'm told is harmless; however, I'm always reluctant to recommend chemicals, particularly if they haven't been used for that long a time. However, if you want a healthy glow, there's nothing wrong with using one of the new skin bronzers that are being marketed by several cosmetic companies. Although bronzers can make you look as if you've just stepped off the beach, they're a lot kinder to your skin. Some even offer UV protection.

PROTECTIVE CLOTHING

A dark T-shirt or slacks will help protect against UV rays. In addition, special SPF outdoor clothing is available at sporting good stores or through mail order.

SUNGLASSES

Sunglasses can prevent squinting, which can promote crow's-feet and fine lines around the eyes. (They can also protect against cataracts.) Be sure to buy sunglasses that offer UV protection.

Dry Skin

Dry, itchy skin is a common complaint among older people, especially in the winter. Dry skin is caused by a reduction in sebum, an oil that forms a protective coating on the skin, thus sealing in moisture. Although you can't replace lost moisture—as some advertisements for skin care products would have you believe—you can bolster the body's own protective seal by using products that reduce water loss from the skin's surface. There are numerous creams and potions on the market that can help seal moisture in. I recommend using fragrance-free, allergy-tested products that don't contain mineral oil, which can deplete the skin of vitamins. Aloe vera creams and lotions and jojoba oil (from the jojoba plant) are excellent for dry skin and are relatively inexpensive. In severe cases, your physician may prescribe a more potent moisturizer.

There are several new-generation moisturizers on the market that contain fancy-sounding compounds such as cholesterol isosterate, ceramides, hyaluronic acid, and fatty acids such as petrolatum and glycolic acid (fruit acids). Basically, despite the hype, these products are similar to traditional moisturizers in that they seal in moisture. However, some may work better than others. There's a wide range of prices among these product lines, and some of the cheaper ones sold at your local drug store may be just as effective as some of the products sold in fancy department stores. Keep in mind that a recent *Consumer Reports* study found that their testers often rated the cheaper skin products higher than the more expensive ones.

Avoid using harsh soaps: soap-free cleaners work well and are far less irritating for most people. Don't bathe or shower in very hot water. An oatmeal bath (Aveeno makes an excellent one) can offer instant relief for dry skin.

Dry heat in particular may sap needed moisture from your skin. Turn off the heat and wear a sweater, or use a humidifier, which can reduce dryness. However, make sure that you are scrupulous about maintaining and cleaning the humidifier because it could be a breeding ground for bacteria and fungi.

For severe dry skin, try taking 1 flaxseed oil capsule three times daily. Within a month, you should see softer, more supple skin.

Cosmeceuticals

Cosmeceuticals refers to a new breed of skin products that offer both therapeutic and cosmetic benefits. Unlike traditional makeups that merely cover up flaws and blemishes, cosmeceuticals contain biologically active ingredients that (at least according to their manufacturers) actually change the quality of the skin. Even skeptics agree that these new breeds of skin creams do have an effect on the outer layers of skin, at least temporarily. Tretinoin (marketed as Retin-A) was the first cosmeceutical. Although originally designed to treat acne, dermatologists noticed that Retin-A appeared to erase fine lines and peeled off the top layer of skin, leaving a pinkish, healthy glow. However, many patients found Retin-A to be very irritating, and it also caused excessive sun sensitivity. Nevertheless, Retin-A is now one of the most prescribed medications in the world. There are also a slew of other cosmeceuticals on the market, notably vitamin A derivatives, alpha-hydroxy acids, salicylic acid, and antioxidants.

RETINOL AND RETINYL PALMITATE

These nonprescriptive-strength vitamin A creams are being touted as antiwrinkle creams without the side effects of Retin-A. Many dermatologists are dubious that these creams are strong enough to be effective; however, they may work well for some people.

ALPHA-HYDROXY ACIDS

Alpha-hydroxy acids (AHAs), which include fruit acid, lactic acid, and glycolic acid, are actually exfolients, that is, they peel dead cells off the surface of the skin, making skin look smoother and less wrinkled. AHAs also help the skin to maintain moisture. Regular use of AHAs can give the skin a fresh glow. Unlike conventional face creams, AHAs are believed to work below the surface of the skin, dissolving the glue that holds the skin together. Over-the-counter products contain between 2 and 10 percent concentrations of AHAs. Dermatologists and plastic surgeons use much stronger concentrations of AHAs in facial skin peels. There is a great deal of controversy regarding the effectiveness and safety of these products. Not all dermatologists agree that AHAs are as effective as their manufacturers say they are. Many contend that over-the-counter products are really not strong enough to have any effect. Some dermatologists worry that the skin will eventually adjust to the AHA and that higher and higher concentrations may be required for any noticeable change. As it stands now, many people find that even low levels of AHAs can be irritating. In addition, some doctors express concern about potential hazards resulting from the long-term use of these new products. They point out that no one knows what, if any, ill affects could arise after several decades of use. What's even more alarming is that some skin salons offer AHA treatments using concentrations of up to 70 percent, which could cause damage. My advice is, proceed with caution. I don't believe that using the lower concentrations of AHAs (under 10 percent) will be harmful as long as you can tolerate it. If you develop any irritation, discontinue the product. Unless the label says otherwise, do not apply an AHA product near the eyes.

SALICYLIC ACID

Similar to AHAs, salicylic acid also sloughs away dead cells and promotes cell turnover (the production of new cells). Salicylic acid may be less irritating for some people, and some dermatologists believe that it is somewhat more effective. At least one study suggested that it promoted faster cell regeneration than AHAs.

ANTIOXIDANTS

Antioxidants are substances that can prevent damage caused by free radicals, unstable oxygen molecules that can destroy healthy cells. UV light in particular can wreak havoc on the skin by creating more of these troublesome free radicals. Antioxidant vitamins such as beta-carotene, E, and C and superoxide dismutase, an antioxidant enzyme that is produced by the body, are included in many skin care products. Although not everyone is convinced of the effectiveness of the external use of antioxidants, it seems plausible that they may help to prevent UV damage. In addition, some researchers believe that antioxidant creams may help to prevent skin cancer.

Chapter 8

A Guide to Commonly Prescribed Drugs

Growing older in the United States has become synonymous with taking pills. Consider the following:

- A study performed at Johns Hopkins University of patients in an ambulatory clinic who were over sixty showed that the typical patient was taking 6.1 drugs simultaneously—4.9 were prescription drugs and the rest were over-the-counter medications. About 25 percent of the patients reported experiencing unpleasant side effects from one or more drugs. About 25 percent of all patients in the study did not even know why the drug or drugs had been prescribed!
- Another study recently published in *The Journal of the American Medical Association* found that close to 25 percent of all Americans over sixty-five were given prescrip-

292 Earl Mindell's Anti-Aging Bible

tions for medications that were either unsafe or ineffective for the elderly. In many cases, side effects resulting from drug interactions or inappropriate medication were dismissed by both patients and their physicians as the normal aches and pains of aging.

Ironically, despite the barrage of drugs, older Americans are none the better for it. In fact, many are worse off. Many of the drugs that are routinely prescribed for older people are not designed for an aging body and often interact badly with other medications. In addition, many of the problems commonly associated with the elderly, such as dizziness, confusion, and weakness, are often caused by the very medication that is supposed to make them healthy! In my opinion, many of the ailments that the elderly are commonly treated for could easily be managed through natural alternatives, such as herbal remedies, diet, and changes in lifestyle.

People of any age should wary of popping pills indiscriminately, but this is particularly true for people over fifty. As we age, our bodies react differently to drugs. An impaired digestive system can interfere with drug absorption. A slowing down of liver and kidney function can lead to problems with breaking down and eliminating a drug, which can cause a toxic buildup. Memory or vision problems or other physical ailments could be affected by medication. Therefore, it is critical for older people to be very wary of taking any medication without first asking specific questions, such as:

What is this medication for?
Can this medication interact with any other medication that I am taking?
Do I have any other medical problem that could be adversely affected by this medication?
Are you giving me the lowest possible dose?
Is this medication safe and effective for a person my age?
What are the side effects?
Do I discontinue the drug or reduce the dose if I experience any side effects?

Are there any alternatives to this medication?
Do I take this drug with food or on an empty stomach?

It is my hope that a healthy lifestyle can eliminate the need for drugs. However, I recognize that it is sometimes necessary to take medication, and the right medication at the right time can indeed be a lifesaver. As a pharmacist, however, I believe that no more than three drugs should be taken simultaneously to avoid interactions or side effects, and that includes over-the-counter medications. If you must take several drugs simultaneously, be sure that you are being closely monitored by your physician.

I have compiled a list of the top thirty drugs prescribed for older people, detailing their potential side effects. Although some of these side effects are rare, I feel it is important for you to know about them. If you do experience any difficulties with medicine, you should notify your doctor immediately. I also discuss possible drug interactions with foods or other drugs, and whenever possible, I recommend natural alternatives. However, if you are taking any prescription medications, do not discontinue your medication for any reason without first checking with your physician. Do not substitute these natural alternatives for your medication unless you are under the supervision of a physician or natural healer.

(Drugs are listed alphabetically by their generic names followed by their common trade names.)
SOURCE: *Physician's Desk Reference*, 1995.

Allopurinol (Zyloprim)

Facts. Prescribed for the treatment of gout.

Possible Side Effects. Skin rashes, hives, itching, fever, headaches, dizziness, drowsiness, nausea, vomiting, diarrhea, stomach cramps, loss of hair from head, chills, joint pains, swollen glands, kidney damage, inflammation of the liver, seizures.

Diet Tips. Watch your vitamin C intake—2 grams (2000 milligrams) of vitamin C can acidify the urine and possibly increase kidney stone formation when used with this drug. Follow a low-purine diet. (See p. 204.)

Caution: Allopurinol can increase the effectiveness of azathioprine and mercaptopurine. It can also thin the blood. When taken with ampicillin, it can cause a skin rash. If you experience drowsiness from this drug, beware of driving or operating heavy machinery.

Personal Advice. Try drinking 1 cup of cherry juice daily to control gout.

Alprazolam (Xanax)

Facts. Mild tranquilizer used to treat anxiety and nervousness.

Possible Side Effects. Drowsiness, light-headedness, headaches, dizziness, fatigue, blurred vision, dry mouth, confusion, hallucinations, depression, excitability, agitation, allergic rash or hives, nausea, vomiting, diarrhea.

Diet Tips. Avoid caffeine, alcohol, and tobacco. Take extra calcium and magnesium, tyrosine, and L-phenylalanine.

Caution: This drug can be addictive. It should not be discontinued abruptly if taken for more than 4 weeks. When taken with digoxin, it can produce toxicity. Smoking may reduce its effectiveness. Other drugs such as levodopa can reduce its effectiveness.

Personal Advice. Exercise is a great stress reliever. Take B vitamins with extra pantothenic acid. Herbs such as passionflower, valerian, hops, skullcap, and chamomile can help reduce tension.

Ambien (Zolpidem)

Facts. Sleep aid.

Possible Side Effects. Drowsiness, dizziness, headaches, nausea, vomiting, amnesia, drug dependency.

Diet Aids. A cup of warm milk or chamomile tea before bedtime can help. Avoid caffeinated beverages and alcohol.
Caution: Do not take other sleep-inducing drugs at the same time as ambien. Be careful of over-the-counter drugs when taking ambien.

Personal Advice. Try using melatonin, valerian, hops, passionflower, skullcap, and calcium and magnesium, which are all natural sleep aids.

Atenolol (Tenormin)

Facts. Used as a treatment for angina and high blood pressure.

Possible Side Effects. Lethargy, fatigue, cold hands and feet, slow heart rate, light-headedness, dizziness, insomnia, abnormal dreams, indigestion, nausea, vomiting, constipation, diarrhea, edema (retention of fluid), joint and muscle discomfort, mental depression, anxiety, chest pain, shortness of breath, decreased libido in both sexes, and impaired erection in men.

Diet Tips. Avoid too much salt. Do not drink alcoholic beverages.
Caution: Do not smoke when taking this drug. Avoid becoming overly heated or overly cold. Be careful when driving or operating heavy machinery. Avoid overexertion. Do not stop drug abruptly; a gradual decrease over 2 to 3 weeks is recommended. This drug can increase the effects of other high blood pressure medications. Monitor closely when taken with insulin. Several drugs can alter the effectiveness of this

drug; check with your physician or pharmacist before taking any other medications.

Personal Advice. Garlic(fresh or supplements), an increase in potassium-rich foods, decrease in sodium, a calcium–magnesium supplement, and celery can help control blood pressure naturally.

Beclomethasone (Vanceril)

Facts: Used to treat asthma.

Possible Side Effects. Fungal infections, skin rashes, dry mouth, sore throat, allergic reactions.

Diet Tips. Check with your physician to make sure that food allergies are not aggravating your condition.

Caution: Do not smoke with this drug. Certain medications including epinephrine (commonly found in cold and allergy medications) can increase the effectiveness of this drug. Check with your physician or pharmacist before using any medications in conjunction with this drug.

Personal Advice. Ephedra tea (also called ma huang) may help with asthmatic symptoms. Use only as directed. If abused, this herb can cause serious side effects including fatal arrhythmias. If you have asthma, do not self-medicate. Consult with a physician or a skilled natural healer.

Captopril (Capoten)

Facts. Treatment for high blood pressure.

Possible Side Effects. Skin rash; swelling of face, hands, and feet; fever; loss of or altered taste; mouth and tongue sores; palpitations; decreased male libido.

Diet Tips. Watch your salt intake. Do not use salt substitutes with potassium or a potassium supplement with this drug unless recommended by your physician. Do not use with alcohol. Food sensitivity may occur with this drug.

Caution: Captopril and potassium could cause serious heart rhythm problems. Captopril can interact poorly with several drugs. Aspirin can decrease effectiveness of captopril. Check with your physician or pharmacist before taking other medications.

Personal Advice. I also recommend eating garlic, losing weight, and reducing your salt intake.

Cimetidine (Tagamet)

Facts. Used to treat peptic ulcers.

Possible Side Effects. Skin rashes, hives, fever, headaches, dizziness, weakness, blurred vision, fatigue, muscular pain, diarrhea, kidney damage, liver damage, agitation, confusion, delirium, hallucinations, slowed heart rate, abnormal bleeding or bruising, decreased libido, impotency, decreased male erection, male breast enlargement, female breast enlargement with milk production.

Diet Tips. Eat a low-protein diet (protein increases stomach acid production). Take a vitamin B_{12} supplement (sublingual or intranasal).

Caution: Citmetidine increases the effectiveness of blood thinners, which can cause internal bleeding. Citmetidine can increase the effectiveness of several other drugs, so check with your pharmacist or physician before taking any other medication. Do not smoke marijuana while using this drug.

Personal Advice. Most specialists feel that an antibiotic is the treatment of choice for this condition, although it is still underprescribed for ulcers. If you are taking cimetidine, ask about antibiotic therapy. In addition, try papayas (whole fruit or tablets), bananas, and a good digestive enzyme. Potato juice, aloe vera juice, and acidophilus capsules may also help relieve symptoms. Marshmallow herb is a time-honored treatment for ulcers.

Conjugated Estrogens (Premarin)

Facts. Estrogen replacement therapy.

Possible Side Effects. Bloating, swelling, and tenderness of the breasts; tan spots on face; skin rashes; hives; itching; headaches; nervous tension; irritability; migraine; depression; stroke.

Diet Tips. Eat foods such as tofu and rye, which are rich in phytoestrogens.

Caution: Be careful about taking estrogen with warfarin (an anticoagulant). Several drugs can adversely react with estrogen. Check with your physician or pharmacist before taking any other medication.

Personal Advice. For relief from menopausal symptoms, try using evening primrose oil, dong quai, vitex, and calcium and magnesium.

Diazepam (Valium)

Facts. Anti-anxiety, anti-alcohol withdrawal symptoms, antiseizure, muscle relaxer.

Possible Side Effects. Drowsiness, lethargy, unsteadiness, rash or hives, dizziness, fainting, blurred or double vision, sweating, nausea, liver damage, low platelet count, bone marrow depression, fever, sore throat, anger, rage, menstrual irregularities, male impotency, inhibition of orgasm in women.

Diet Tips. Restrict coffee, colas, and other caffeinated beverages. Do not use with alcohol.

Caution: Heavy smoking may reduce the effectiveness of this drug. Do not use with marijuana. Do not drive or attempt any hazardous activity while taking this drug. Be careful about overheating your body while taking this drug. Do not discontinue abruptly. Taper off dosage to prevent unpleasant withdrawal. Digoxin and phenytoin may decrease the effectiveness of this drug. Several other drugs including cimeditine and oral contraceptives may increase the drug's effectiveness. Check with your physician or pharmacist before using this drug with another medication.

Personal Advice. A B-complex vitamin, calcium and magnesium, valerian, hops, passionflower, and chamomile would greatly decrease the need for this drug.

Digoxin (Lanoxin, Lanoxicaps)

Facts. Heart stimulant used in congestive heart failure that helps to maintain normal heart rate and rhythm.

Possible Side Effects. Headaches; drowsiness; confusion; blurred or yellow-green vision; nausea; vomiting; diarrhea; allergic reactions, including skin rashes or hives; decreased libido; impotency; breast enlargement in males.

Diet Tips. Eat potassium-rich foods including potatoes, canteloupe, and bananas. Avoid caffeinated drinks. Don't smoke tobacco or marijuana.

Caution: Do not take diuretics (water pills) or quinine. Many drugs are synergistic (can increase the effectiveness) with digoxin, such as ibuprofen, captopril, and indomethacin. Check with your physician or pharmacist before taking any other medication, either prescription or over the counter.

Personal Advice. Herbs such as hawthorne berries and cayenne are cardiotonics. Vitamins and supplements including vitamin E, coenzyme Q_{10}, and L-carnitine, which can strengthen the heart muscle, help metabolize fats and dissolves blood clots.

Diltiazem (Cardizem)

Facts. Used to treat angina and high blood pressure.

Possible Side Effects. Fatigue, light-headedness, changes in heart rate and rhythm, palpitations, skin rashes, hives, itching, headaches, drowsiness, dizziness, nervousness, insomnia, depression, confusion, hallucinations, nausea, indigestion, constipation, male impotence.

Diet Tips. Avoid too much salt. Do not use with alcohol.
Caution: Do not smoke tobacco or marijuana when using this drug. When taken with beta-blockers or digitalis drugs, diltiazem can cause heart rhythm disorders. Cimeditine increases the diltiazem's effectiveness.

Personal Advice. Garlic, celery, calcium and magnesium, passionflower, valerian, a B-complex vitamin, coenzyme Q_{10}, hawthorn berries, vitex.

Dyazide (Hydrochlorothiazide and Triamterene)

Facts. A diuretic used to treat congestive heart failure.

Possible Side Effects. High potassium blood level, low sodium level, low blood pressure, dehydration, discolored urine, skin rash, itchiness, headaches, dizziness, unsteadiness, weakness, drowsiness, lethargy, dry mouth, nausea, vomiting, diarrhea, anaphylactic shock, confusion numbness, tingling of lips and face, slow heart rate, shortness of breath.

Diet Tips. Do not increase intake of potassium-rich foods or take potassium supplements while taking this drug. Avoid salt substitutes containing potassium. Do not use this drug if you are nursing. Drink alcohol with caution or not at all.

Caution: Avoid taking with captopril, indomethacin, and lithium. Amantadine and digoxin can increase the effectiveness of this drug. Withdraw from this drug slowly. If you are over sixty, take this drug for 2 to 3 weeks and then check with your physician to make sure it is working properly. Dehydration (loss of body fluid) can occur, which can lead to stroke, heart attack, and thrombophlebitis. Do not operate heavy machinery if dizziness or drowsiness occurs. This drug can cause sensitivity to sunlight.

Personal Advice. Weight loss, exercise, garlic, and calcium and magnesium can help reduce the need for this drug.

Enalapril Maleate (Vasotec)

Facts. Used to treat high blood pressure.

Possible Side Effects. Dizziness; light-headedness; fainting; skin rashes; fatigue; itching; headaches; nervousness; numbness; tingling; rapid heart rate and palpitations; digestive disorders; excessive sweating; muscle cramps; swelling of face, tongue, and vocal chords; abnormal bleeding; bruising.

Diet Tips. Do not use salt substitutes while taking this drug without first checking with your physician; they usually contain potassium, which can cause serious complications when taken with enalapril maleate. Salt intake should be adjusted by your physician. Alcohol consumption should be moderated.

Caution: Avoid potassium supplements; they can cause serious heart rhythm disturbances when taken with this drug. Enalapril maleate combined with certain drugs can also lead to dangerously high potassium levels. Do not take any medications without first checking with your physician or

302 Earl Mindell's Anti-Aging Bible

pharmacist. **Do not overheat your body; blood pressure can drop precipitously, causing serious effects when using this drug.**

Personal Advice. Weight loss, salt restriction, garlic (fresh or supplements), calcium and magnesium, and celery can go a long way to reduce the need for this drug.

Fluoxetine Hydrochloride (Prozac)

Facts. Used to treat depression.

Possible Side Effects. Decreased appetite, weight loss, skin rash, hives, itching, headaches, dizziness, fatigue, difficulty concentrating, changed taste, nausea, vomiting, diarrhea, seizures, weakness, fever, joint pain, fluid retention, dry mouth, impaired erection or orgasm, suicidal tendencies.

Diet Tips. Do not use with alcohol.
Caution: Do not drive if this drug causes drowsiness. Prozac increases the effectiveness of digitalis drugs, coumadin (an anticoagulant), antidiabetic drugs, and other monoamine oxidase inhibitors, including meperidine hydrochloride and phenelzine sulfate.

Personal Advice. Tyrosine, taurine, L-phenylalanine, B-complex, and exercise can reduce the need for this drug.

Flurazepam Hydrochloride (Dalmane)

Facts. A short-term treatment for insomnia.

Possible Side Effects. Hangover upon rising, drowsiness, lethargy, unsteadiness, skin rash, hives, burning eyes, tongue swelling, dizziness, fainting, blurred vision, double vision, slurred speech, nausea, indigestion, nervousness, irritability, apprehension, euphoria, excitement, hallucinations, impaired white blood cell production, liver damage, sore throat, fever.

Diet Tips. Caffeine should be restricted within 4 hours of taking this drug. Do not use with alcohol.

Caution: This drug may be habit forming with long-term use. Smoking heavily will decrease the effectiveness of flurazepam hydrochloride. Do not use marijuana while taking this drug. If you are over sixty, use the smallest possible dose to avoid overdose. Don't drive or operate heavy machinery while taking this drug. Do not discontinue drug abruptly. Flurazepam hydrochloride can increase the effectiveness of digoxin and phenytoin; I would not advise taking these drugs together. Flurazepam hydrochloride can decrease the effectiveness of levodopa, cimetidine, birth control pills, and other drugs. Check with your pharmacist or physician before taking flurazepam hydrochloride with other drugs.

Personal Advice. A calcium and magnesium supplement, passionflower, hops, valerian, and exercise can greatly reduce the need for this drug.

Furosemide (Fumide, Lasix)

Facts. A diuretic used for congestive heart failure, high blood pressure with other medication. Increases calcium excretion.

Possible Side Effects. Skin rashes, hives, fever, headaches, blurred vision, ringing in the ears, numbness, tingling, fatigue, weakness, digestive complaints, jaundice, abnormal bleeding or bruising, impotence in men, can increase the likelihood of diabetes, gout, and drug-induced lupus.

Diet Tips. Diuretics can sap your body of important minerals including potassium. Eat a high-potassium diet including bananas, potatoes, cantaloupe, and plain yogurt. Decrease salt intake to prescribed amount. Watch all processed food for sodium content. Watch your drinking: alcohol and furosemide can cause blood pressure to drop too low.

Caution: Be careful of sun exposure: some people develop photosensitivity (sensitivity to sunlight). Beware of interactions with many other drugs, including digoxin and indomethacin. If you are over sixty, start with a very small dose until your response can be determined. Too high a dosage can lead to stroke, heart attack, or vein inflammation with a blood clot.

Personal Advice. To reduce your need for this drug take a calcium–magnesium or garlic supplement. Chew on celery stalks. Drink lots of water. Eat fresh dandelion leaves or take dandelion root capsules. Vitamin B_6 is also a natural diuretic.

Ibuprofen (Advil, Motrin, Rufen)

Facts. Treatment for moderate or severe pain, available over the counter in doses of 200 milligrams. Prescription strengths also available at 400, 600, and 800 milligrams per tablet or capsule.

Possible Side Effects. Fluid retention, discolored urine, skin rash, hives, itching, headache, dizziness, blurred vision, ringing in ears, depression, mouth sores, indigestion, nausea, vomiting, constipation, diarrhea, severe skin reactions, peptic ulcers, liver damage, kidney damage, menstruation irregularities, male breast enlargement and tenderness, mild anemia, suppressed bone marrow.

Diet Tips. Do not use with alcohol.
Caution: Drive with caution. Ibuprofen can increase the effectiveness of acetaminophen and anticoagulant medicines. Check with your physician or pharmacist before taking ibuprofen with other drugs.

Personal Advice. Try the amino acid D,L-phenylalanine and white willow bark for moderate pain control.

Lorazepam (Ativan)

Facts. Used to treat anxiety.

Possible Side Effects. Sedation, dizziness, weakness, unsteadiness, disorientation, depression, nausea, change in appetite, headaches, sleep disturbances, agitation, vision problems, rashes.

Diet Tips. Do not use with alcohol. Restrict caffeinated beverages.

Caution: Heavy smoking may reduce the effectiveness of this drug. Do not use with marijuana. Do not drive or attempt any hazardous activity while taking this drug. Be careful about overheating your body while taking this drug. Do not discontinue abruptly. Taper off dosage to prevent unpleasant withdrawal. Digoxin and phenytoin may decrease the effectiveness of this drug. Several other drugs including cimetidine and birth control pills may increase the drug's effectiveness. Check with your physician or pharmacist before using this drug with another medication.

Personal Advice. A B-complex vitamin, calcium and magnesium, valerian, hops, passionflower, and chamomile would greatly decrease the need for this drug.

Lovastatin (Mevacor)

Facts. Used to treat high cholesterol.

Possible Side Effects. Abnormal liver function, skin rashes and itching, headaches, dizziness, blurred vision, digestive disturbances, nausea, muscle pain, cataracts, bleeding ulcers.

Diet Tips. Eat a low-fat diet with no more than 20 percent of calories from fat. Avoid saturated fat.

Personal Advice. Vitamins E and C, garlic, psyllium, charcoal, yogurt, pectin, and oat bran can reduce the need for this drug.

Metoprolol (Toprol XL)

Facts. Used to control mild to moderate blood pressure.

Possible Side Effects. Lethargy, fatigue, cold hands and feet, slow heart rate, light-headedness, dizziness, insomnia, abnormal dreams, indigestion, nausea, vomiting, constipation, diarrhea, edema (retention of fluid), joint and muscle discomfort, mental depression, anxiety, chest pain, shortness of breath, decreased libido, impaired erection.

Diet Tips. Avoid too much salt. Do not use with alcohol.
Caution: Do not smoke when taking this drug. Avoid becoming overly heated or overly cold. Be careful when driving or operating heavy machinery. Avoid overexertion. Do not stop drug abruptly; a gradual decrease of 2 to 3 weeks is recommended. Metoprolol tartrate can increase the effects of other high blood pressure medications. Monitor closely when taken with insulin. Several drugs can either increase or reduce the effectiveness of this drug. Check with your physician or pharmacist before taking any other medication.

Personal Advice. Garlic (fresh or supplements), an increase in potassium-rich foods, decrease in sodium, a calcium–magnesium supplement, and celery can help control blood pressure naturally.

Naproxen (Naprosyn)

Facts. Pain reliever, anti-inflammatory.

Possible Side Effects. Fluid retention, prolonged bleeding time, skin rash, hives, itching, localized swelling, spontaneous bruising, headaches, dizziness, nausea, vomiting, abdominal pain, diarrhea, inhibited evacuation (one report), menstrual irregularities.

Diet Tips. Do not use with alcohol.

Caution: Naproxin can increase the effectiveness of acetaminophen and anticoagulants such as coumadin and can increase bleeding with aspirin and other drugs. Be sure to check with your pharmacist or physician if you are taking this drug with other medication.

Personal Advice. D,L-phenylalanine, white willow bark, quercetin, and bromelin are also good pain relievers and anti-inflammatories.

Nifedipine (Procardia)

Facts. Used to treat angina and mild to moderate high blood pressure.

Possible Side Effects. Low blood pressure, rapid heart rate, swelling of feet and ankles, flushing, sweating, skin rash, hives, itching, fever, headaches, dizziness, weakness, nervousness, blurred vision, palpitations, shortness of breath, wheezing, coughing, heartburn, nausea, abdominal cramps, diarrhea, tremors, muscle cramps, altered menstrual cycle, excessive menstrual flow.

Diet Tips. Avoid excess salt. Do not use with alcohol.

Caution: Do not smoke tobacco or marijuana. Do not overheat yourself. Do not stop taking this drug cold turkey; gradually taper drug off under a physician's supervision.

Personal Advice. Try using hawthorn berries, garlic, cayenne, calcium and magnesium, hops, valerian, and chamomile.

Piroxicam (Feldene)

Facts. Prescribed for mild to severe pain and inflammation.

Possible Side Effects. Fluid retention, prolonged bleeding time, skin rash, itching, bruising, headaches, dizziness, blurred vision, ringing in the ears, drowsiness, fatigue, difficulty concentrating, nausea, vomiting, abdominal pain, diarrhea, peptic ulcers, ulcerative colitis, mild anemia.

Diet Tips. Do not use with alcohol.
Caution: Piroxicam can increase the effectiveness of acetaminophen and anticoagulants. Do not drive when taking this drug. Check with your doctor or pharmacist before using piroxicam with other drugs.

Personal Advice. D,L-phenylalanine, white willow bark, fish oil, quercetin, and bromelin can be used instead of piroxicam.

Propanolol Hydrochloride (Inderal)

Facts. Used to treat angina and high blood pressure and to prevent migraine headaches.

Possible Side Effects. Lethargy, fatigue, cold hands and feet, slow heart rate, light-headedness, dizziness, insomnia, abnormal dreams, indigestion, nausea, vomiting, constipation, diarrhea, edema (retention of fluid), joint and muscle discomfort, mental depression, anxiety, chest pain, shortness of breath, decreased libido, impaired erection in men.

Diet Tips. Avoid too much salt. Do not use with alcohol.
Caution: Do not smoke when taking this drug. Avoid becoming overly heated or cold. Be careful when driving or operating heavy machinery. Avoid overexertion. Do not stop drug abruptly; a gradual decrease of 2 to 3 weeks is recommended. This drug can increase the effects of other high

blood pressure medications. Monitor closely when taken with insulin. Several drugs can alter the effectiveness of this drug; check with your physician or pharmacist before taking any other medications.

Personal Advice. Garlic (fresh or supplements), an increase in potassium-rich foods, decrease in sodium, a calcium–magnesium supplement, and celery can help control blood pressure naturally.

Ranitidine Hydrochloride (Zantac)

Facts. Used to treat ulcers.

Possible Side Effects. Skin rash, headaches, dizziness, feeling ill, nausea, drowsiness, constipation, diarrhea, confusion in elderly, hepatitis, bone marrow depression, weakness, sore throat, bruising, decreased libido, male impotency, breast enlargement in men.

Diet tips. Do not use with alcohol. Ranitidine hydrochloride can increase your blood alcohol concentration by 34 percent. Talk to your physician about a special diet. A high-protein diet can increase stomach acid secretions, which can worsen your condition.
Caution: Be cautious when using ranitidine hydrochloride with anticoagulant; it can increase the risk of bleeding. This drug can make you drowsy. Be careful when driving or operating heavy machinery.

Personal Advice. Most specialists feel that an antibiotic is the treatment of choice for this condition, although it is still underprescribed for ulcers. If you are taking ranitidine hydrochloride, ask about antibiotic therapy. In addition, try papayas (whole fruit or tablets), bananas, and a good digestive enzyme. Potato juice, aloe vera juice, and acidophilus capsules may also help relieve symptoms. Marshmallow herb is a time-honored treatment for ulcers.

Terfenadine (Seldane)

Facts. Antihistamine.

Possible Side Effects. Dry nose, mouth, and throat; skin rash; itching; headache; nervousness; fatigue; increased appetite; indigestion; nausea; vomiting; swollen breasts in women.

Diet Tips. None.
Caution: Do not use this drug with ketoconazole. Check with your physician or pharmacist before taking this drug with other medications.

Personal Advice. Try ephedra tea or ma huang. Use only the prescribed dose. If abused, this herb can cause serious side effects including fatal arrhythmias.

Theophylline (Theo-Dur)

Facts. Anti-asthmatic and bronchodilator

Possible Side Effects. Nervousness, insomnia, rapid heartbeat, increased urination, skin rashes, hives, headaches, dizziness, irritability, tremors, fatigue, weakness, loss of appetite, nausea, vomiting, abdominal pain, diarrhea, excessive thirst, flushing in the face.

Diet Tips. Do not have caffeine with this drug.
Caution: This drug can interact adversely with several drugs. For example, it decreases the effectiveness of lithium and phenytoin (which means you may require a higher dose) and increases the effectiveness of allopurinol and oral contraceptives (which means you may require a lesser dose). Check with your pharmacist or physician before using theophylline with any over-the-counter or prescription drug.

Triamcinolone Acetonide (Azmacort)

Facts. Used to treat bronchial asthma.

Possible Side Effects. Yeast infections of mouth and throat; irritations of mouth, tongue, and throat; skin rash; swelling of face; hoarseness; cough.

Diet Tips. Check to see if food allergies could be worsening your condition.
Caution: Albuterol, ephedrine hydrochloride, terubaline, and theophylline may increase the effectiveness of this drug.

Personal Advice. Try ephedra tea or ma huang. Use only the prescribed dose. If abused, this herb can cause serious side effects including fatal arrhythmias. Asthma should be treated by a physician or skilled healer.

Triazolam (Halcion)

Facts. Short-term treatment for insomnia.

Possible Side Effects. Drowsiness, dizziness, light-headedness, euphoria, tachycardia, fatigue, confusion, memory impairment, abdominal cramps, pain, depression, visual disturbances.

Diet Tips. Do not use with alcohol. Restrict caffeinated beverages.
Caution: Heavy smoking may reduce the effectiveness of this drug. Do not use with marijuana. Do not drive or attempt any hazardous activity while taking this drug. Be careful about overheating your body while taking this drug. This drug can be habit forming. Do not discontinue abruptly; taper off dosage to prevent unpleasant withdrawal. Digoxin and phenytoin may decrease the effectiveness of this drug. Several other drugs including cimetidine and oral contraceptives may

increase the drug's effectiveness. Check with your physician or pharmacist before using this drug with another medication.

Personal Advice. Melatonin, calcium and magnesium, hops, passionflower, and valerian are also good for insomnia.

Verapamil Hydrochloride (Calan)

Facts. Used to treat angina, high blood pressure, and heart rhythm irregularities.

Possible Side Effects. Low blood pressure, fluid retention, skin rash, hives, itching, aching joints, headaches, dizziness, fatigue, nausea, indigestion, constipation, menstrual irregularities, male breast enlargement and impotency.

Diet Tips. Avoid too much salt. Do not use with alcohol.
Caution: Do not smoke tobacco or marijuana when taking this drug. Verapamil can increase the effectiveness of carbamazepine and digoxin. When taken together with beta-blockers, this drug can affect heart rhythm. Cimetidine can increase the effectiveness of verapamil.

Personal Advice. Garlic (fresh or supplements), celery, calcium and magnesium, passionflower, hops, valerian, a B-complex vitamin, hawthorn berries, vitex, coenzyme Q_{10} are also excellent for lowering blood pressure.

Selected Bibliography

Acoustic Neuroma Association Notes, no. 36 (December 1990).

Adlercreutz, Herman. "Plasma Concentrations of Phyto-Oestrogens in Japanese Men." *The Lancet* 342 (November 13, 1993): 1209–1210.

———. "Lignans and Phytoestrogens: Possible Protective Role in Cancer." *Frontiers of Gastrointestinal Research* 14 (1988): 165–176.

Adlercreutz, H., E. Hamalainen, S. Gorbach, and B. Goldin. "Dietary Phyto-oestrogens and the Menopause in Japan. *Lancet* 339 (May 16, 1992): 1233.

"Aloe Update." *The Lawrence Review of Natural Products* 3 no. 21 (November 15, 1982).

Anderson, James W. "Dietary Fiber and Diabetes." *Journal of the American Dietetic Association* 87, no. 9 1189–1197 (September 1987).

———. *The HCF Guide Book.* Lexington, Ky: HCF Diabetes Foundation, 1987.

Armstrong, S. M., and J. R. Redman. "Melatonin: A Chronobiotic with Anti-Aging Properties." *Medical Hypotheses* 43 (1991): 300–309.

Aspirin as a Therapeutic Agent in Cardiovascular Disease. Dallas, Tex.: American Heart Association, 1993.

Balch, James F., and Phyllis A. Balch. *Prescription for Nutritional Healing.* Garden City, N.Y.: Avery Publishing Group, 1990.

Barbul, Adrian, et al. "Arginine Stimulates Lymphocyte Immune Response in Healthy Human Beings." *Surgery* 90, no. 1 (1981): 244–251.

Be Your Best: Nutrition After Fifty. Washington, D.C.: American Institute for Cancer Research, 1988.

"Beyond Deficiency: New Views on the Function and Health Effects of Vitamins." Howerde E. Sauberlich and Lawrence T. Muchlin, eds. *The New York Academy of Sciences* (February 9–12, 1992) (abstracts).

Bitterman, Wilhelm A., et al. "Environmental and Nutritional Factors Significantly Associated with Cancer of the Urinary Tract Among Different Ethnic Groups." *Urologic Clinics of North America* 18, no. 3 (August 1991).

Bland, Jeffrey. *Bioflavonoids: The Friends and Helpers of Vitamin C in Many Hard-to-Treat Ailments.* New Canaan, Conn.: Keats Publishing Inc., 1984.

Block, Gladys, Donald E. Henson, and Mark Levine, eds. "Ascorbic Acid: Biologic Functions and Relation to Cancer." Proceedings of the National Institutes of Health, Bethesda, Md., September 10–12, 1990. *American Journal of Clinical Nutrition* 54, no. 6 (suppl.) (December 1991).

"Blocking Skin Cancer Through Diet?" *Tufts University Diet and Nutrition Letter* 12, no. 5 (July 1994).

Blumenthal, Mark. "Echinacea Highlighted as Cold and Flu Remedy." *Herbalgram*, no. 29 (1993): 8–9.

"Borage Seed Oil and Evening Primrose Oil May Relieve Arthritis Pain and Swelling." *Environmental Nutrition* (March 1994).

Borum, Peggy R. "Carnitine." *Annual Review in Nutrition* 3 (1983): 233–259.

Bowman, Barbara. "Acetyl-Carnitine and Alzheimer's Disease." *Nutrition Reviews* 50, no. 5. 142–143.

Bradlow, H. Leon, and Jon Michnovicz. "A New Approach to the Prevention of Breast Cancer." *Proceedings of the Royal Society of Edinburgh* 95B (1989): 77–86.

Brody, Jane. "Folic Acid Emerges as a Nutritional Star." *New York Times,* March 1, 1994.

Bunce, George Edwin. "Nutritional Factors in Cataract." *Annual Review of Nutrition* 10 (1990): 223–254.

" . . .But Study of Women Finds Iron May Contribute to Higher Coronary Disease Risk." *News from the American Heart Association,* (June 13, 1994).

Burtin, Ritva B., Carolyn Clifford, and Elaine Lanza. "NCI Dietary Guidelines: Rationale." *American Journal of Clinical Nutrition* 48 (1988): 888–895.

Butterworth, C. E., et al. "Folate Deficiency and Cervical Dysplasia." *Journal of the American Medical Association* 267, no. 4. 528–533 (January 22/29, 1992).

Cancer Facts and Figures—1993. Atlanta, Ga: American Cancer Society, 1993.

Caragay, Alegria B. "Cancer-Preventive Foods and Ingredients." *Food Technology* 46, no. 4 (April 1992): 65–68.

Castleman, Michael. "Red Pepper Is Hot!" *Medical Selfcare* (September/October 1989): 68–69.

Cerda, J. J., et al. "The Effects of Grapefruit Pectin on Patients at Risk for Coronary Heart Disease Without Altering Diet or Lifestyle." *Clinical Cardiology* 11, no. 9 (September 1988): 589–594.

Chen, K.J., and Chen, K. "Ischemic Stroke Treated with Ligusticum chuanxiong." *Chinese Medical Journal* 105, no. 10 (October 1992): 870–873.

Chinthalapally, Rao V., et al. "Inhibitory Effect of Caffeic Acid Esters on Azoxymethane-Induced Biochemical Changes and Aberrant Crypt Foci Formation in Rat Colon." *Cancer Research* 53 (September 15, 1993): 4182–4188.

"Chronic Stress is Directly Linked to Premature Aging of the Brain." *National Institute on Aging, Research Bulletin* (October 1991).

Cutler, Richard G. "Antioxidants and Aging." *American Journal of Clinical Nutrition* 53 (1991): 373S–379S.

Darlington, L. Gail. "Dietary Therapy for Arthritis." *Rheumatic Disease Clinics of North America* 17, no. 2 (May 1991): 273–285.

Darlington, L. G., and S. W. Ramsey. "Clinical Review: Review of Dietary Therapy for Rheumatoid Arthritis." *British Journal of Rheumatology* 32 (1993): 507–514.

Devi, P.U., et al. "In Vivo Inhibitory Effect of *Withania somnifera* (Ashwagandha) on a Transplantable Mouse Tumor, Sarcoma 180." *Indian Journal Experimental Biology* 30, no. 3 (March 1992): (169–172).

Diet and Cancer. Washington, D.C.: American Institute for Cancer Research, Information Series, 1992.

Diet, Nutrition, and Prostate Cancer. Washington, D.C.: American Institute for Cancer Research, Information Series, 1991.

Dizziness, Hope Through Research. U.S. Department of Health and Human Services, National Institutes of Health, September 1986.

"Do Monounsaturated Fats and Vitamin E Provide Double-Barreled Protection Against Coronary Ills?" *News from the American Heart Association* (April 11, 1994).

Dorgan, Joanne F., and Arthur Schatzkin. "Antioxidant Micronutrients in Cancer Prevention." *Hematology/Oncology Clinics of North America* 5, no. 1, 43–68.

Duke, James A. "An Herb a Day: Clubmoss, Alias Lycopodium Alias

Huperzia." *Business of Herbs* (January/February 1989).

Elegbede, J. A., et al. "Regression of Rat Primary Mammary Tumors Following Dietary d-Limonene." *Journal of the National Cancer Institute* 76, no.2 (February 1986): 323–325.

"Estrogen and Alzheimer's." *Harvard Women's Health Watch* 1, no. 11 (July 1994).

Evans, W. J. "Exercise, Nutrition and Aging." *Symposium: Nutrition and Exercise, Journal of Nutrition* 122: 796–801, 1992.

"Exercise and Arthritis: The Importance of a Regular Program." *University of California, Berkeley, Wellness Letter* (April 1994).

"Exercise in 90-Year-Olds Increases Muscle Strength and Mobility." *National Institute on Aging Research Bulletin* (September 3, 1990).

Fackelmann, K.A. "Chicken Cartilage Soothes Aching Joints." *Science News* (September 25, 1993): 198.

———. Do EMFs Pose Breast Cancer Risk?" *Science News* 45 (June 18, 1994): 145.

———. "Nutrients May Prevent Blinding Disease." *Science News Letter* 145 (September 12, 1994).

"Facts and Fiction About Memory Aging: A Quantitative Integration of Research Findings." *Journal of Gerontology* 48, no. 4 (1993): 157–171.

Facts on Prostate Cancer. Atlanta, Ga.: American Cancer Society, 1988.

Feldman, Henry A., et al. "Impotence and Its Medical and Psychosocial Correlates: Results of the Massachusetts Male Aging Study." *Journal of Urology* 151 (January 1994): 54–61.

Fiatarone, Maria, Evelyn F. O'Neill, and Nancy Doyle Ryan. "Exercise Training and Nutritional Supplementation for Physical Frailty in Very Elderly People." *New England Journal of Medicine* 330, no. 25. 1769–1775 (June 23, 1994).

"Flax Facts." *Journal of the National Cancer Institute* 83, no. 15 (September 7, 1991): 1050–1052.

"The Food Guide Pyramid." *Department of Agriculture, Home and Garden Bulletin,* no. 252 (August 1992).

Garland, Cedric F., Frank C. Garland, and Edward D. Gorham. "Can Colon Cancer Incidence and Death Rates Be Reduced with Calcium and Vitamin D?" *American Journal of Clinical Nutrition* 54 (1991): 193S–201S.

"Garlic Fights Nitrosamine Formation . . . as Do Tomatoes and Other Produce." *Science News* 145 (1991): 190.

"Ginger and Atractylodes as an Anti-inflammatory." *Herbalgram,* no. 29 (1993): 19.

Giovannucci, Edward, Eric B. Rimm, and G. Colditz. "A Prospective Study of Dietary Fat and Risk of Prostate Cancer." *Journal of the National Cancer Institute* 85, no. 19. 1571–1579 (October 16, 1993).

Graf, Ernst, and John W. Eaton. "Antioxidant Functions of Phytic Acid." *Free Radical Biology and Medicine* 8 (1990): 61–69.

Hackman, Robert M. "Palm Oil Carotene: An Exciting New Innovation in Nutrition Supplementation." *Whole Foods* (December 1993).

Heart and Stroke Facts. Dallas, Tex.: American Heart Association.

Heimburger, D.C., et al. "Improvement in Bronchial Squamous Metaplasia in Smokers Treated with Folate and Vitamin B_{12}: Report of a Preliminary Randomized, Double-Blind Intervention Trial." *Journal of the American Medical Association* 259, no. 10 (March 11, 1988): 1525–1530.

"Herbs and Spices May be Barrier Against Cancer, Heart Disease." *Environmental Nutrition* 16, no. 6 (June 1993).

al-Hindawi, M. K., S.H. al-Khafaji, and M.H. Abdul-Nabi. "Antigranuloma Activity of Iraqi Withania Somnifera." *Journal of Ethnopharmacology* 37, no. 2 (September 1992): 113–116.

Hobbs, Christopher, and Steven Foster. "Hawthorne: A Literature Review." *Herbalgram*, no. 22, (Spring 1990): 19–33.

Hocman, Gabriel. "Prevention of Cancer: Vegetables and Plants." *Comparative Biochemistry and Physiology* 93B, no. 2 (1989): 201–212.

Hodge, Marie. "Immunity Breakthrough: The 6000-Year-Old Rx." *Longevity* (January 1993).

Horwitt, Max K. "Therapeutic Uses of Vitamin E." *Resident and Staff Physician* (December 1982): 38–46.

Horwitz, Crystal, and Alexander R.P. Walker. "Lignans—Additional Benefits from Fiber?" *Nutrition and Cancer* 6, no. 2 (1984): 73–76.

How Men Stay Young. Emmaus, Pennsylvania: Rodale Press, 1991.

"Improved Physician/Patient Communication Can Minimize Some Drug Side Effects." *National Institute on Aging Research Bulletin*, (January 30, 1989).

"In Vino Veritas—and Something for Your Heart." *Heartstyle* 4, no. 3 (summer 1994).

Jaakkola, K., et al. "Treatment with Antioxidants and Other Nutrients in Combination with Chemotherapy and Irradiation in Patients with Small-Cell Lung Cancer." *Anticancer Research* 12 (1992): 599–606.

Jain, Adesh K., et al. "Can Garlic Reduce Levels of Serum Lipids? A Controlled Clinical Study." *American Journal of Medicine* 94 (June 1993): 632–635.

Johnson, Kathleen, and Evan W. Kligman. "Preventive Nutrition: An 'Optimal' Diet for Older Adults." *Geriatrics* 47, no. 10 (1992): 56–60.

Johnston, Carol S., Claudia Meyer, and J.C. Srilakshmi. Vitamin C Elevates Red Blood Cell Glutathione in Healthy Adults." *American Journal of Clinical Nutrition* 58 (1993): 103–105.

Joosten, Etienne, et al. "Metabolic Evidence That Deficiencies of Vitamin B_{12} (Cobalamin), Folate, and Vitamin B_6 Occur Commonly in Elderly People." *American Journal of Clinical Nutrition* 58 (1993): 468–476.

Kamikawa, Todashi, et al., "Effects of Coenzyme Q_{10} on Exercise Tolerance in Chronic Stable Angina Pectoris." *American Journal of Cardiology* 56 (1985): 247–251.

Khachaturian, Zaven S. "Calcium and the Aging Brain: Upsetting a Delicate Balance?" *Geriatrics* 46, no. 6, 78–79, 83 (1991).

Khan, A. et al. "Insulin Potentiating Factor and Chromium Content of Selected Foods and Spices." *Biologic Trace Element Research* 24, no. 3 (March 1990): 183–188.

Kravitz, Howard M., Hector C. Sabelli, and Jan Fawcett. "Dietary Supplements of Phenylalanine and Other Amino Acid Precursors of Brain Neuroamines in the Treatment of Depressive Disorders." *Journal of the AOA* 84, no. 1 119–123 suppl. (September 1984).

Kune, Gabriel, Susan Bannerman, and Barry Field. "Diet, Alcohol, Smoking, Serum ß-carotene and Vitamin A in Male Nonmelanocytic Skin Cancer Patients and Controls." *Nutrition and Cancer* 18, no. 3 (1992): 237–244.

Lee, H. P., L. Gourley, and S.W. Duffy. "Dietary Effects on Breast-Cancer Risk in Singapore." *Lancet* 337 (May 18, 1991): 1197–1200.

Leighton, Terrance, Charles Ginther, and Larry Fluss. "The Distribution of Quercetin and Quercetin Glycosides in Vegetable Components of the Human Diet." Paper presented at the Royal Society of Chemistry Conference, September 1992.

Lipkin, Richard. "Wine's Chemical Secrets." *Science News* 144, (October 23, 1993): 264–265.

"Long-Distance Runners Double 'Dilating' Capacity of Their Coronary Arteries, Researchers Find." *News from the American Heart Association,* (April 12, 1993).

Mabey, Richards, ed. *The New Age Herbalist.* New York: Collier Books, 1988.

"Magnesium Lowers Blood Pressure in Some Diabetic Hypertensives." *News from the American Heart Association,* (September 13, 1990).

"Major Study Reports 'Huge' Variance in Heart Rates Among Nations." *News from the American Heart Association,* (July 11, 1994).

McCaleb, Rob. "Astralagus." *Herb Research Foundation* (July 30, 1990).

———. "Bilberry: Microcirculation Enhancer." *Herb Research Foundation* (April 29, 1992).

McKeown-Eyssen, Gail E., and Elizabeth Bright-See. "Dietary Factors in Colon Cancer: International Relationships." *Nutrition and Cancer* 6, no. 3 (1984).

McMurdo, Marion E. T. and Lucy Rennie. "A Controlled Trial of Exercise by Residents of Old People's Homes." *Age and Ageing* 22 (1993): 11–15.

Meydani, M., et al. "Protective Effect of Vitamin E on Exercise-Induced Oxidative Damage in Young and Older Adults." *American Journal of Physiology* 264 (*Regulatory Integrative Comparitive Physiology* 33) (1993): R992–998.

Michnovicz, Jon J., and H. Leon Bradlow. "Induction of Estradiol Metabolism by Dietary Indole 3-Carbinol in Humans." *Journal of the National Cancer Institute* 82, no. 11. 947–949 (June 6, 1990).

"Mining for Minerals—Zinc is Worth Its Weight in Gold." *Environmental Nutrition* 17, no. 9 (September 1994).

"Mining for Toxic Minerals Hidden in Our Diets." *Environmental Nutrition* 15, no. 3 (March 1992).

Moriguchi, Satori, et al. "Functional Changes in Human Lymphocytes and Monocytes After in Vitro Incubation with Arginine." *Nutrition Research* 7 (1987): 719–728.

National Institute on Aging, Research Bulletin, (February 20, 1990).

National Institute on Aging, Research Bulletin, (April 1991).

National Institute on Aging, Research Bulletin, (July 1991).

National Institute on Aging, Research Bulletin, (October 1991).

National Institute on Aging, Research Bulletin, (August 1992).

National Institute on Aging, Research Bulletin, (November 1992).

Negri, Eva, Carlo La Vecchia, and Silvia Francheschi. "Vegetable and Fruit Consumption and Cancer Risk." *International Journal of Cancer* 48 (1994): 350–354.

Nelson, Miriam E., Elizabeth C. Fisher, and Avraham F. Dilmanian. "A 1-Year Walking Program and Increased Dietary Calcium in

Postmenopausal Women: Effects on Bone." *American Journal of Clinical Nutrition* 53 (1991): 1304–1311.

Newsome, D. A., et al. "Oral Zinc in Macular Degeneration." *Archives of Ophthalmology* 106, no. 2 (February 1988): 192–198.

"Niacin: Double-Edged Sword for Lowering Cholesterol." *Tufts University Diet & Nutrition Letter* 12 no. 6 (August 1994).

Nielson, Forrest H. "Studies on the Relationship Between Boron and Magnesium Which Possibly Affects the Formation and Maintenance of Bones." *Magnesium Trace Elements* 9 (1990): 61–19.

————. "Ultratrace Minerals Mythical Elixirs or Nutrients of Concern?" *Biologic Association of Medicine of Puerto Rico* 83 (1981): 131–133.

"NIH Consensus Development Conference: The Treatment of Sleep Disorders in Older People." *National Institute on Aging Research Bulletin* (September 3, 1990).

1995 Heart and Stroke Facts Statistics. Dallas, Tex.: American Heart Association.

Nixon, Daniel W., Myron Winick, and Michelle Maher. "Metabolic Efficiency, Energy Intake, and Cancer." *Cancer Prevention* 1, no. 3 (1991).

"No Need for Kidney Stone Sufferers to Curb Calcium." *Environmental Nutrition* (September 1993).

"Noise and Hearing Loss, Consensus Statement." *NIH Consensus Development Conference* 8, no. 1 (January 22–24, 1990).

Odens, Max. "Prolongation of the Life Span in Rats." *Journal of the American Geriatrics Society* 21, no. 10 (1973): 450–451.

"On the Link Between Diet and Gout." *Tufts University Diet & Nutrition Letter* 10, no. 9 (November 1, 1992).

Packer, Lester. "Protective Role of Vitamin E in Biologic Systems." *American Journal of Clinical Nutrition* 53 (1991): 1050S–1055S.

Panush, Richard S. "Does Food Cause or Cure Arthritis?" *Rheumatic Disease Clinics of North America* 17, no. 2 (May 1991): 259–271.

Penn, N.D., et al. "The Effect of Dietary Supplementation with Vitamins A, C, and E on Cell-Mediated Immune Function in Elderly Long-Stay Patients: A Randomized Controlled Trial." *Age and Ageing* 20 (1991): 169–174.

Perchellet, J.P., et al. "Antitumor-Promoting Activities of Tannic Acid, Ellagic Acid, and Several Gallic Acid Derivatives in Mouse Skin." *Basic Life Sciences* 59 (1992): 783–801.

Peto, R., et al. "Can Dietary Beta-Carotene Materially Reduce Human Cancer Rates?" *Nature* 290 (March 1981): 201–207.

Press, Raymond I., Jack Geller, and Gary Evans. "The Effect of Chromium Picolinate on Serum Cholesterol and Apolipoprotein Fractions in Human Subjects." *The Western Journal of Medicine* 152, no. 1 (January 1990): 41–45.

"Preventing Wintertime Bone Loss: Effect of Vitamin D Supplementation in Healthy Postmenopausal Women." *Nutrition Reviews* 50, no. 2 (February 1992): 52–54.

"Preventive Nutrition: Disease-Specific Dietary Interventions for Older Adults." *Geriatrics* 47, no. 11 (November 1992): 39–49.

"Prostate Cancer and Red Meat." *University of California, Berkeley, Wellness Letter* (February 1994).

Pryor, William A. "Can Vitamin E Protect Humans Against the Pathological Effects of Ozone in Smog? *American Journal of Clinical Nutrition* 53 (1991): 702–722.

"Pumping Immunity." *Nutrition Action Healthletter* (April 1993).

Raloff, Janet. "Hearty Vitamins: Sparing Arteries with Megadose Supplements." *Science News* 142 (1991): 78.

Regan, T. J. "Alcohol and the Cardiovascular System." *Journal of the American Medical Association* 264, no. 3 (1990): 377–381.

"Reviving Your Taste Buds When Taste and Smell Wane." *Enviromental Nutrition* (February 1993).

Risch, Harvey A., et al. "Dietary Factors and the Incidence of Cancer of the Stomach." *American Journal of Epidemiology* 122, no. 6 (1985).

Robertson, James McD., Allan P. Donner, and John R. Trevithick. "A Possible Role for Vitamins C and and E in Cataract Prevention." *American Journal of Clinical Nutrition* 53 (1991): 346S–351S.

Roe, Daphne, A. "Overview of Effects of Aging on Nutrition." *Clinics in Geriatric Medicine* 6, no. 2 (May 1990): 319–334.

Roebothan, Barbara Vera, and Ranja Kuma Chandra. "Relationship between Nutritional Status and Immune Function of Elderly People." *Age and Ageing* 23 (1994): 49–53.

Rose, David P. "Diet, Hormones and Cancer." *Annual Review of Public Health* 14 (1993): 1–17.

———. "Dietary Fiber, Phytoestrogens, and Breast Cancer." *Nutrition* 8, no. 1 (January/February 1992): 47–51.

Rosenberg, Irwin H., and Joshua W. Miller. "Nutritional Factors in Physical and Cognitive Functions of Elderly People." *American Journal of Clnical Nutrition* 55, (1992): 1237S–1243S.

Rusting, Ricki L. "Why Do We Age?" *Scientific American* 267, 1 (December 1992): 131–141.

Sandyk, Reuven. "Possible Role of Pineal Melatonin in the Mechanisms of Aging." *International Journal of Neuroscience.* 52 (1990): 85–92.

Schardt, David. "Alzheimer's in the Family." *Nutrition Action Health-letter* (June 1994).

Schmidt, Karlheinz. "Antioxidant Vitamins and ß-Carotene: Effects on Immunocompetence." *American Journal of Clinical Nutrition* 53 (1991): 383S–385S.

"Seedy Remedy for Rheumatoid Arthritis?" *Science News* 144 (November 6, 1993): 302.

Selkoe, Dennis J. "Aging Brain, Aging Mind: Structural and Chemical Changes." *Scientific American* 267, no. 3 (September 1992).

Sharma, Om P., et al. "Soy of Dietary Source Plays a Preventive Role Against the Pathogenesis of Prostatitis." *Journal Steroid Biochemical Molecular Biology* 43, no. 65 (1992): 557–564.

Shephard, Roy J. "Exercise and Aging: Extending Independence in Older Adults." *Geriatrics* 48, no 5. 61–64 (May 1993).

Siani, Alfonso, et al. "Increasing the Dietary Potassium Intake Reduces the Need for Antihypertensive Medication." *Annals of Internal Medicine* 115 (1991): 753–759.

Simopoulos, Artermis P. "Omega-3 Fatty Acids in Health and Disease and in Growth and Development." *American Journal of Clinical Nutrition* 54 (1991): 438–463.

Smigel, Kara. "Vitamin E Moves on Stage in Cancer Prevention Studies." *Journal of the National Cancer Institute* 84, no. 13 (July 1, 1992).

Snyder, Jessica. "Solving the Alzheimer's Jigsaw." *Longevity* (January 1992).

Soni, K.B., A. Rajan, and R. Kuttan. "Reversal of Aflatoxin Induced Liver Damage by Turmeric and Curcumin." *Cancer Letter* 66, no. 2 (September 30, 1992): 115–121.

"Staying Physically Active May Help to Stave Off Blood Vessel Ills, Two New Studies Suggest." 33rd Annual Conference on Cardiovascular Disease Epidemiology and Prevention. *News from the American Heart Association* 18 (Abstract 17).

Stern, Yaakov, et al. "Influence of Education and Occupation on the Incidence of Alzheimer's Disease." *Journal of the American Medical Association* 271, no. 13 (April 6, 1994).

Tanaka, T., et al. "Inhibition of 4-Nitroquinoline-1-oxide-Induced Rat Tongue Carcinogenesis by the Naturally Occurring Plant Phenolics Caffeic, Ellagic, Chlorogenic and Ferrulic Acids." *Carcinogenesis* 14, no. 7 (July 1993): 1321–1325.

Teas, Jane. "The Consumption of Seaweed as a Protective Factor in the Etiology of Breast Cancer." *Medical Hypotheses* 7 (1981): 601–613.

Teel, R.W., and A. Castonguay. "Antimutagenic Effects of Polyphenolic Compounds." *Cancer Letter* 66, no. 2 (September 30, 1992): 107–113.

"A Test to Take (and Not to Take) for Colon Cancer." *University of California, Berkeley, Wellness Letter* 9, no. 12 (September 1993).

Thun, Michael J., et al. "Risk Factors for Fatal Colon Cancer in a Large Prospective Study." *Journal of the National Cancer Institute* 84, no. 19. 149–1500(October 7, 1992).

"Triglycerides Finally Unmasked as 'Bad Actor' in Coronary Artery Disease Drama, Researchers Say." *News from the American Heart Association,* (July 1994).

Troll, Walter, and Ann R. Kennedy, eds. "Workshop Report from the Division of Cancer Etiology, National Cancer Institute, National Institutes of Health. Protease Inhibitors as Cancer Chemopreventive Agents." *Cancer Research* 49 (January 15, 1989): 499–502.

Tucker, Don M., et al. "Nutrition Status and Brain Function in Aging." *American Journal of Clinical Nutrition* 52 (1990): 93–102.

"23-Year Study of Middle-Aged Men in Hawaii Confirms: Physical Activity Will Lower Risk of Heart Disease." *News from the American Heart Association,* (June 13, 1994).

U.S. *Department of Agriculture, Food and Nutrition, Research Briefs* Washington, D.C. (January–March 1993).

U.S. *Department of Agriculture, Food and Nutrition, Research Briefs* (July–September 1993).

U.S. Department of Agriculture, Human Nutrition Research Center on Aging at Tufts University, Research Program Description.

U.S. *Department of Agriculture, Research Briefs* (April–June 1993).

Varma, Shambhu D. "Scientific Basis for Medical Therapy of Cataracts by Antioxidants." *American Journal of Clinical Nutrition* 53 (1991): 335–345S.

"Vitamin B_6 and Immune Function in the Elderly and HIV-Seropositive Subjects." *Nutrition Reviews* 50, no. 5 (May 1992): 145–147.

"Vitamin E May Guard Against Artery Blockage by LDL." *Heartstyle* (Fall 1993).

"Vitamin E Supplementation Enhances Immune Response in the Elderly." *Nutrition Reviews* 50, no. 3 (March 1992): 85–87.

Walsh, Nicolas E., et al. "Anagesic Effectiveness of D-Phenylalanine in Chronic Pain Patients." *Archives of Physical Medicine Rehabilitation* 67 (July 1986): 436–439.

Wei-Hua, Lu, Jiang Shou, and Xi-Can Tang. "Improving Effect of Huperzine A on Discrimination Performance in Aged Rats and Adult Rats with Experimental Cognitive Impairment." *Acta Pharmacologica Sinica* 1 (January 1988): 11–15.

Wuethrich, B. "Higher Risk of Alzheimer's Linked to Gene." *Science News*, 144 (August 14, 1993).

You, W.C., et al. "Allium Vegetables and the Reduced Risk of Stomach Cancer." *Journal of the National Cancer Institute* 81, no. 2 (1989): 162–164.

Ziegler, Regina G. "Vegetables, Fruits, and Carotenoids and the Risk of Cancer." *American Journal of Clinical Nutrition* 53 (1991): 251S–259S.

Znaiden, Alex. "The Science Behind Successful New Skin Care Products." *Avanstar Communications* (January 1994).

Index